The Clinical Problem of Masochism

The Clinical Problem of Masochism

Edited by Deanna Holtzman, PhD,
and Nancy Kulish, PhD

ROWMAN & LITTLEFIELD
Lanham • Boulder • New York • London

Published by Rowman & Littlefield
A wholly owned subsidiary of The Rowman & Littlefield Publishing Group, Inc.
4501 Forbes Boulevard, Suite 200, Lanham, Maryland 20706
www.rowman.com

Unit A, Whitacre Mews, 26-34 Stannery Street, London SE11 4AB

British Library Cataloguing in Publication Information Available

Library of Congress Cataloging-in-Publication Data
The hardback edition of this book was previously cataloged by the Library of Congress as
follows:

The clinical problem of masochism / edited by Deanna Holtzman and Nancy Kulish
p. cm.
Includes bibliographical references and index.
I. Holtzman, Deanna. II. Kulish, Nancy. [DNLM: 1. Masochism—physiopathology. 2.
Masochism—psychology.WM610]
616.85'835—dc23
2012029911

ISBN 978-0-7657-0860-1 (hardback : alk. paper)
ISBN 978-1-4422-4297-5 (pbk. : alk. paper)
ISBN 978-0-7657-0861-8 (electronic)

♾™ The paper used in this publication meets the minimum requirements of American
National Standard for Information Sciences—Permanence of Paper for Printed Library
Materials, ANSI/NISO Z39.48-1992.

Printed in the United States of America

To David and Harold

Contents

Acknowledgments   ix

Introduction: The Suffering of Sisyphus   1
Deanna Holtzman, PhD, and Nancy Kulish, PhD

1   Clinical Constellations of Masochistic Psychopathology   15
Otto F. Kernberg, MD

2   Masochism in Childhood and Adolescence as a Self-Regulatory Disorder   29
Alan Sugarman, PhD

3   Some Suggestions for Engaging with the Clinical Problem of Masochism   51
Kerry Kelly Novick and Jack Novick, PhD

4   Clinical Observations on Masochistic Character Structure   77
Robert Alan Glick, MD

5   Sadomasochistic Stuckness   89
Stanley J. Coen, MD

6   Masochism as a Multiply-Determined Phenomenon   103
Glen O. Gabbard, MD

7   Self-Abuse and Suicidality: Clinical Manifestations of Chronic Narcissistic Rage   113
Anna Ornstein, MD

8   Varieties of Masochistic Experience: Modes of Analytic Relating   129
Henry Markman, MD

9   Masochism and Trauma   145
Harold P. Blum, MD

10   Failure to Thrive: Shame, Inhibition, and Masochistic Submission in Women   161
Dianne Elise, PhD

11   Analysts Who Have Sexual Relations with Their Patients: The Central Role of Masochism   187
Marvin Margolis, MD, PhD

Conclusion 197
    Deanna Holtzman, PhD, and Nancy Kulish, PhD
Index 199
About the Contributors 207

Acknowledgments

This book grew from and was inspired by an ongoing discussion group at the American Psychoanalytic Association on masochism. We want to thank all of the presenters and the participants over the years who generously shared clinical experiences and stimulating questions that led to the clinical focus of this book.

Special thanks are owed to Karen Holtzman for her expertise in doing background research and editing this volume. She made our work much easier.

Introduction:
The Suffering of Sisyphus

Deanna Holtzman, PhD, and Nancy Kulish, PhD

Sisyphus, the legendary king of Corinth, was condemned by Zeus to perpetually push a huge boulder up a hill, which when it reached the top, inevitably rolled down again. This story captures the experience of working with masochistic patients. They present us with their lives in which they, like Sisyphus, relentlessly suffer. Horowitz (1990) writes about a masochistic patient whose history was replete with self-punishing failures and disastrous relationships, The patient, after years of prior analyses and beginning a third analysis, angrily likened himself to Sisyphus. In trying to help such patients, we, too, feel like Sisyphus. They seem chained to suffering—indeed to seek it out—and to resist change which would make their lives better. We, as clinicians, often begin to feel hopeless and defeated.

Masochistic phenomena are found in individuals across the diagnostic spectrum of individuals who frequent the offices of clinicians. Certainly, they pose the most perplexing, serious and "resistant-to change" therapeutic challenges. This book is an attempt to address these clinical difficulties. To that end, we have asked highly respected clinicians and theoreticians, who have made major contributions to psychoanalytic understandings of masochism, to share their ideas with us about how they actually work with masochistic patients. Each of our contributors demonstrates that clinicians, working within broadened conceptual frameworks and therapeutic approaches, can now better help masochistic patients. Each of our authors enhances the diagnostic and conceptual scope of masochistic phenomena. Each asserts that masochistic phenomena are solutions to psychological and emotional problems. Each emphasizes the entrenched nature of problems of masochism as well as the inextricable and invariable presence of sadism as a major part of the picture. (Thus we will refer to masochism but bear in mind the concept always refers to sadomasochism.) And finally, each author documents the arduous, lengthy and troubling nature of such treatments with the inevitably intense countertransferences that are aroused. But, as our readers will see, their creative and pragmatic approaches will give hope and help in dealing with these symptoms, behaviors and character issues which are so familiar to all working in the various fields of mental health. The readers will instantly recognize the clinical pictures of sadomasochistic dilemmas in the clinical situation and hopefully glean ideas as to how to deal more effectively with these phenomena.

THE CLINICAL PROBLEM OF MASOCHISM: THEORETICAL BACKGROUND

The clinical problem of masochism is a daunting one that has been with psychoanalysis since the beginning. For Freud (1924), masochism posed thorny conceptual problems and contradictions for his developing theories of the instincts and of the pleasure principle. At the same time, Freud spoke to the clinical problem of masochism, in the context of bringing an end to an analysis in "Analysis Terminable and Interminable" (1937): "for the moment we must bow to the superiority of the forces against which we see our efforts come to nothing. Even to exert a psychical influence on simple masochism is a severe tax upon our powers" (p. 243).

Contemporary psychoanalysts who struggle to understand and to help such patients rely in part on many of the concepts left to us by Freud (1905, 1919, 1924): his definition of masochism—pain as a condition for pleasure; the intimate relationship of masochism and sadism, paired first as component instincts; masochism resulting from turning the aggressive drive from an object outside the self onto the self; the importance of unconscious guilt, especially related to the oedipal situation; and finally, as a manifestation of the enigmatic death drive.

Parallel to general developments in the field, contemporary psychoanalysts have both enhanced and deepened these approaches to the treatment of masochism. A first major shift has been from Freud's instinctual theories to a focus on early object relationships and narcissism. Masochism (or sadomasochism) is seen, from varying theoretical vantage points, as a characterological or neurotic response to early narcissistic injuries, and/or to early losses, deprivations and other trauma. For example, one idea is that a masochistic relationship is experienced as better than no relationship at all, or that pain must be suffered in order to keep the early object tie, or represents a struggle to take control over the painful loss of early omnipotence (Novick and Novick, 1987, 1991; Cooper, 2009) or also to master and claim victory over calamity and trauma (Ellman, 2009). From a vantage point of self-psychology, masochism is understood as a means of repairing a faulty or fragile self or as a means of holding a fragmenting sense of self together in the midst of fragmentation (Ornstein, as cited in Cooper and Sacks, 1991; Goldberg, 1993). Sadomasochistic behavior is also seen as a means of affect regulation (Grotstein, 1984) or as the manifestation of identification with powerful, hated parental imagos (Gabbard, 2000). From a Kleinian perspective, comes the description of "enthrallment" in a masochistic addiction or drive toward death (Joseph, 1982). Not all still hold to Freud's early definition; some deemphasize the sexual aspect (Cooper, 1988). Many analysts, however, retain the original importance allotted to the erotic in masochism: by analyzing the defensive and adaptive functions of sexualization (Goldberg, 1993; Kernberg, 1991; Coen, 1981) or examining the sexualized sadomasochistic tie to the object on whom one is pathologically dependent (Coen, 1992). In this book, the reader will find many of these sorts of understandings elaborated and brought to life in the clinical examples.

A second major shift in the scrutiny of masochism has been from the one-person model to a two-person model, from the early explorations of its meanings in the patient's psychic economy to the analyst's participation in a shared (sado)masochistic experience and to an exploration of the total transference/countertransference picture. In their clinical approaches, contemporary analysts rely heavily on and let themselves be guided by their often tortured countertransference reactions to their masochistic patients, to the see-saw of critical, frustrated or sadistic responses to the interplay of helpless, terrified, pain-ridden states of mind that fill the consulting room. Kleinians track the shifting projective identifications of such feelings; self-psychologists use their empathic attunement to the patient's pain as a way to illuminate the dark crevices of the difficult analytic process; postmodern Freudians stay attuned to the sadomasochistic enactments played out in the analytic dyad.

These major shifts in theory and technique will be illustrated by our contributors. In 1988, Glick and Meyer provided an excellent and comprehensive review of the literature on masochism up to that time. Since then, our contributors have been in the forefront in taking up where the review left off. While drawing upon Freud, Klein, Cooper, Bion, Lacan, British object-relationists, and neo-Kleinians, they all bring fresh insights based on their clinical experiences to contemporary understandings of masochism.

The major focus of this book is clinical and pragmatic. Each contributor, in different ways, focuses on the challenging clinical dilemmas posed by masochism. The reader will find vivid and clear clinical examples and explanations of how particular theoretical views lead to new understandings and specific interventions in treatments designed to alleviate the misery that these patients suffer and bring about.

CONTEMPORARY UNDERSTANDINGS OF MASOCHISM

Definition and Diagnosis

All of the contributors in this book seem to agree on a broadened definition of masochism, without the obligatory sexual component proposed by Freud. Ornstein, for example, suggests adopting a working definition of masochism as a term loosely denoting phenomena in which suffering, submission or defeat are prominent or tenacious and seem driven or self-induced. Blum puts it simply as consciously or unconsciously seeking pain, suffering and humiliation. Kernberg gives us an excellent framework and overview of the clinical manifestations of masochism. He argues that the specific diagnosis—that is, the subgroup of type of masochistic disorder—determines any prognostic and therapeutic implications. What is most important clinically, and what will determine the efficacy of treatment, is the organization of the underlying personality structure. He starts his description of the various "clinical constellations" defining masochism, from the most pathological, severe perversions (loss of life and limb) through the more neurotic-like personality structures (such as moral masochism). He clearly and carefully documents the differing levels of development underlying the various clinical constellations of masochism. Markman underlines this idea and observes that within the same individual, masochistic phenomena reflect internal object relationships from different developmental levels.

Many frame the definition in terms of inner and outer object relationships, as, for example, the Novicks, who refer to a "relational psychopathology." For Blum, too, it is crucial to look at the level of the person's object relations in evaluating the quality of masochism as well as the meaning of the masochistic behavior. Ornstein evaluates masochism somewhat differently in terms of the qualities of the underlying structures of the self. Notably, Sugarman expands the definition of masochism to include very young children.

The Developmental Origins and Underlying Meanings of Masochism

Each of our authors clearly articulates their views of the underlying meanings, origins and functions of the masochistic phenomena that they encounter in their patients and demonstrate how these understandings inform their clinical work. All stress that there are multi-determinants, meanings, and functions of masochism which need to be interpreted to the patient. Blum, in this vein, stresses the need for multi-disciplinary research on aspects of masochism.

Trauma

Most of our authors agree that trauma of some sort, occurring in early childhood, is what underlies masochistic constellations. This emphasis on the idea of trauma as a precipitating factor in the development of masochism is a major contribution to the psychoanalytic literature on the topic. Blum centers his contribution on trauma as the underlying, although not necessarily unitary or unifying explanation, of masochism. Gabbard, too, writes that masochistic symptoms can be understood as the individual's effort to master early trauma, by for example, unconsciously orchestrating the repetition of childhood trauma. Similarly, the Novicks describe life-long "closed-system" adaptations to trauma, not easily set aside. Glick feels that deprivation, cruelty and psychic abuse in childhood promote the internalization of the idea that one must submit to the other in order to get love and pleasure.

The concept of adjustment to accumulated trauma in development figures predominantly in these accounts. Sugarman describes masochism originating in cumulative trauma in a three-year-old child; Ornstein explains the effects of trauma in the development of masochistic phenomena from a self-psychological explanation. She goes on to say that parental mis-attunement and abuse adversely affect the optimal development of the structures of the self. Accumulated trauma, she suggests, lies in narcissistic wounds stemming from being deprived of legitimate developmental needs for merger and mirroring. Traumatic experiences such as physical, sexual, and verbal abuse generate further narcissistic rage which cannot be voiced in childhood because it could threaten precarious connections to a disappointing, rejecting and abusive environment. In order to assure continued connection to the frustrating and/or abusive caretaker, infants and young children may develop what Bernard Brandschaft (2007) called "pathological accommodations" that function as protection "against intolerable pain and existential anxiety." Sugarman suggests another very important antecedent for future masochism: physical illness in an infant or young child who then cannot be soothed.

Narcissism and Early Object Relations

Following other contemporary thinking, all of the present contributors trace masochism's origins to narcissistic issues and additional aspects of early object relations. Margolis and Gabbard endorse the intimate connection between narcissism and masochism. Coen explicates the patterns of "stuckness" or "pathological dependency" in masochistic patients who cling to their internal objects and to the sadomasochistic relationships in their lives and who are terrified of separation and autonomy for themselves. Thus, change is felt to be an impossibility. Markman clearly elucidates the internal object relations in masochism: the feeling is of being trapped and bound to "bad internal objects" which are persecutory parts of the self. Kernberg, too, emphasizes the internalized aggression. He states that the basic origin of masochism is the internalization of real or fantasied aggression, which then is reflected in the earliest sadistic precursors to the superego. Gabbard shows that patients are as adept at tormenting others as themselves. He underscores the fact that much of the pleasure of masochism comes from taking revenge on parents by defying their expectations.

Elise uses object relations as the basis of understanding the phenomenon of masochistic surrender. According to Elise, the masochistic individual feels she must surrender in order to be accepted by an internal or real object. In other words, the masochistic choice is to submit or to lose connection, to be alone and isolated or to be connected. Elise also links narcissism in the development of masochism via the sense of shame. She outlines a developmental narrative that centers on a bodily-focused narcissistic injury and sense of shame in response to unrequited erotic longings. She concludes that shame is the underside of masochism as well as narcissism.

Similarly, the Novicks present "a developmental tale of masochism." From what they have named "the closed system" of handling early narcissistic difficulties, the individual becomes prone to masochistic solutions which become fixed patterns of relating. In the closed system, the basis for mastery is omnipotent belief in the power and necessity to be a perpetrator or victim in order to survive. Underscoring the close connection between narcissism and masochism that many of the authors accept, Kernberg writes how the masochist, in his suffering, may hold on to an inner sense of narcissistic triumph over those who might wish to help him.

Finally, Glick poses an important, and often neglected, question about inborn factors in masochism: is it the product of a particular form of developmental trauma, or does it reflect, a particular *temperamental* vulnerability of failure of ego structures and self-organization?

From these varying perspectives on the developmental origins of masochism, trauma, narcissistic difficulties, and early object relations, the contributors all approach the clinical problem of masochism asking similar questions: what is the meaning of the masochistic behavior? What functions do clinging to painful relationships serve for the individual? How might the masochistic behavior be a defense against feelings of helplessness or a means of regulating painful affects?

Sexuality, or the Erotic Component of Masochism

Given this emphasis on narcissism and early trauma related to masochism, we might ask: is there still a place for sexuality and the concomitant dynamics in the understanding of masochistic phenomena which have seemingly been pushed into the background in much of the current discussions? Is the concept of libidinalization or sexualization of pain still useful clinically? Can we observe triadic, oedipal constellations as well as, and differentiated from, dyadic, pre-oedipal constellations in masochism?

In observing how these psychoanalysts work with masochistic patients, it seems that sexuality and oedipal dynamics have been pushed into the background while pre-oedipal issues have come to the fore. True, all of the contributors advance the idea that masochistic phenomena are multiply determined and reflect conflicts from *all* levels of development. Gabbard and Kernberg give rich clinical examples that demonstrate this concept, and Kernberg suggests a full examination of the patient's sexual life to determine the existence and/or the level of masochistic pathology. Several describe their work with individuals who suffer sexual masochistic perversions. For example, one of the patients presented by Blum had a kind of sexual perversion with persistent fantasies about being controlled and humiliated by a dominatrix. Blum's interpretations of these compulsions encompassed, in part, oedipal guilt, which led the patient to seek punishment masochistically. At the same time, Blum felt that acute and extended traumas in his patient's infancy and early childhood were the foundation of his later masochistic disposition. Blum then demonstrates how these early problems became a focus in the therapeutic work.

What our authors describe is a complex picture with early narcissistic and troubled object relations then effecting and intermingling with later sexual pleasures. For example, Ornstein describes how sexual abuse leads to narcissistic rage, which in turn is transformed into masochistic behaviors. The Novicks describe how omnipotent fantasies and modes of functioning stemming from early developmental periods make it impossible for the child to enjoy ordinary sexual pleasures of later developmental periods, and then show up in adult patients in masochistic character structures and behaviors. Relying heavily on the work of the Novicks, Sugarman argues that the origins of masochism occur pre-oedipally and that true masochism does exist in young children.

Elise focuses her contribution on oedipal or triadic dynamics which underlie masochistic surrender often found in women. She suggests that the sense of oedipal defeat in girls is double-fold: first, in desiring to win her father, she loses to her rival, her mother; and second, her homoerotic impulses toward the mother, which are also part of the early triangular drama, go unacknowledged and are thus experienced as unacceptable. So it is that a girl's sexuality and sense of self may become organized around a sense of defeat and self-defeating masochism, which then become a typical mode of adaptation. Elise proposes that oedipal defeat in relation to either partner can result in a narcissistic injury experienced and expressed in terms of gender or generational differences. She suggests that the "common masochism of everyday life" often goes under the radar in women's sexual relationships as women foreclose their potential to be potent sexually.

Several of the authors suggest that something else, usually aggression, underlies the sexual manifestations in masochistic phenomena. Coen suggests that "erotization tames destructiveness." Thus, the erotic side of masochistic behavior can serve as a defense against underlying aggression. The Novicks and Blum also explicitly argue that aggression is far more important or basic in masochism than sexuality. Sugarman argues defensive sexualization has contributed to the mistaken notion that "true" masochism is based on oedipal conflicts. But Glick reminds us, importantly, that there is still value in understanding the nature and meaning of unconscious desire. And, tellingly, Margolis evokes the story of *Oedipus Rex* and incestuous desire to help explain sexual boundary violations.

Unconscious Guilt

Another question related to the role of sexuality is: "what is the role of unconscious guilt in masochistic phenomena, and how is it handled clinically?" Unconscious guilt, another conjectured component of masochism, was first advanced by Freud and is utilized by our authors differently in the clinical work illustrated here. The Novicks speak of severe guilt that accompanies the "closed system" or omnipotent character structures involved in masochism. Similarly, Margolis finds masochism organized around sadistic and primitive superego functions.

Kernberg names unconscious guilt from severe superego pressures as one of the major components in definitions and categorizations of masochism. In his chapter, Blum provides a clear review of psychoanalytic understandings about the relationship of unconscious guilt and masochism. He also describes how unconscious oedipal guilt in one of his cases led the individual to punish himself masochistically. While he makes reference to unconscious guilt in his clinical formulations, Glick concludes that the model is insufficient for treating entrenched masochistic character, as does Sugarman.

Ornstein does not conceptualize masochistic dynamics in terms of a compromise formation in which unconscious guilt is supposed to play a particularly important role by simultaneously permitting gratification and punishment for forbidden incestuous sexual wishes, but rather emphasizes underlying trauma (real events) and narcissistic pathology. Both she and Coen emphasize the important idea of the masochistic strategy of inducing the *other* to feel guilt. Ornstein describes how the masochistic patient tries to make others responsible for his suffering and thus indirectly expresses his sadism.

Markman, following the Kleinians, puts it differently. He perceives masochism as a manifestation of the death drive, one clinical manifestation of which is a refusal to face guilt in the depressive position, `a la Melanie Klein. He feels that the death drive, "which annihilates need," is a psychological, not a biological concept. This annihilation involves a turn toward omnipotent fantasy and action, which deny the pain and anxiety of separateness and dependency. The fantasies and actions are destructive and anti-life.

The readers will find that all of these conceptualizations determine the form and focus of the interventions and attitudes in each of the clinical examples.

THERAPEUTIC CONSIDERATIONS

Therapeutic work with sadomasochistic patients, if it is to be at all successful, is described by our authors as long and difficult. There seem to be no fast cures.

Negative Therapeutic Reactions

What about the relationship of masochism and the so-called "negative therapeutic reaction," as described in the literature? Is it in the masochistic patients in whom the true "negative therapeutic reactions" are found? That is, any positive step in the treatment is followed by a Sisyphean step backward, by an undoing of forward progress; the patient cannot let himself succeed. In their own unique and interesting way, each contributor describes this phenomenon and demonstrates the intense resistances to change in masochistic phenomena, what Betty Joseph (1982) has characterized as "a pull toward failure." It is these resistances to change that make the treatments of masochistic patients so "long and arduous," in Glick's words. Several of the authors offer motivations for the negative therapeutic reactions seen in masochistic patients. Glick describes how patients have to keep any tiny success or pleasure secret from the analyst. Blum suggests that the patient's unconscious need to defeat the clinician results in "negative therapeutic reactions," and Kernberg states that deep unconscious guilt in depressive masochistic character may account for negative therapeutic reactions.

Transferences and Countertransferences

For all our authors, the major clinical focus is turned on the transference/countertransference drama that unfolds between the analyst/therapist and the patient. Kernberg, for example, suggests that the systematic and in-depth exploration of the masochistic scenario as it appears in the transference is necessary for any success in the treatment. He reminds us that the working through and resolution of the "pathological grandiose" self is via the transference. Transference/countertransference takes center stage in these treatments because, in some degree, *all* of our authors view masochism as relational pathology in the sense of internal relationships between self and object representations and how these are played out in interpersonal relationships.

Certainly, for all of the authors, the key to working with masochistic patients lies in recognizing and using the intense countertransferences that inevitably arise. Their clinical accounts demonstrate repeatedly how the clinician becomes dismayed and unsettled by feeling unappreciated, defeated, incompetent, helpless and victimized or even murderous. We will see the ways in which our contributors work constructively with these feelings rather than disregard them or allow them to grow and, in the worst case scenario, defeat the treatment or become enacted in boundary violations. We feel this current focus on how to work with the countertransference is a major contribution to the clinical problem of masochism.

Coen admonishes us to learn to tolerate hating and being hated that arise as we are drawn into sadomasochistic struggles. He advises us to let ourselves identify with our patients' shame. He reminds us to try to normalize the intense countertransferences that are always present and advises us to be alert in order to avoid gross enactments. He helps us to understand and thus to help our patients to realize their unconscious wishes to torment us, to recognize the sadism that hides within their masochism and the unconscious pleasure they derive from it. Thinking along the lines of the "stuckness" that Coen describes, Margolis states that analysts who have committed boundary violations in retrospect report feeling stuck in countertransference binds with their patients with whom they have gotten in trouble.

The Novicks describe for us the dramas that mark such treatments, in which the patient's goal is to avoid any change, while the clinician in turn experiences pain, helplessness, and lack of attention. They suggest that the therapist realize that this scenario may be a repetition of an early experience in the patient's life, when the patient was on the receiving end of painful experiences with a caretaker. Becoming aware of this, the clinician may better bear and contain his responses to being rendered helpless.

Similarly, Glick describes being paralyzed by his countertransferences. Tangled up with masochistic patients in their motivated pursuit of suffering, we, too, can become wounded as our efforts appear, at times, to bring further misery to the situation. The inevitable traumatizing object relationship comes alive in the transference/countertransference, and the therapist becomes caught up in the drama, becoming so frustrated that he wants to abandon the patient and thus confirm the patient's expectations.

In working with children, Sugarman describes the specific countertransferences of indignation and frustration that arise in working with sadistic parents.

Emphasis on the "Here and Now"

Clearly, most feel that the center of the work must be played out and dealt with in the crucible of the transference within the immediate present. Markman seems to feel the strongest about this point. He describes in minute detail how he works in the here and now with his patient trying to understand and to get the patient to understand what is happening between them. He asserts that *it is only by carefully analyzing this sadomasochistic structure that is lived out with the analyst that we may eventually find out about the nature of the patient's underlying anxieties, lack of self-cohesion, unconscious fantasies and possible traumatic experiences.* In contrast, Ornstein feels that one can work out, or certainly begin to work out, with the patient the meanings of his or her masochistic behavior outside of the transference. This is in keeping with her idea that the origins of masochism lie in real "lived experiences"—that is, events in the reality of the patient's life. Both Markman and Ornstein, as they listen to their patients, pay close attention to the state of self-esteem.

Paradigm for Marital Dynamics

Elise gives a psychoanalytic orientation to working with couples and helping them extricate themselves from sadomasochistic dynamics. She addresses what she calls a "maso-narcissistic union"—a masochistic-narcissistic relational pairing seen in some heterosexual couples. The backdrop for such a pairing is masochistic surrender in women and a devaluation of the female in men. Instead of organizing her clinical approach in terms of sadomasochism, however, she creatively uses the notion of "a failure to thrive" dynamic. Her interpretative strategy allows the patient not to feel condemned or judged.

Towards a Goal of Self Reflection

Another therapeutic consideration is the importance of trying to get the patient to be more self-reflective, as Markman in particular stresses, to find some distance from suffering and to pull out of the constant tallying of victimhood. Connected to this goal, both Markman and Gabbard also try to help their patients focus on their unconscious motivations and often highly defended yearnings for more connectedness with them. What must stay in the clinician's mind are the questions: "What is the something that the masochistic solution is better than?" and "What is it about?" This question—"What is this about?"—is posed one way or the other, implicitly and often explicitly, to the patient so that the patient can get some distance from the self-induced masochistic suffering. Markman, in particular, advocates not looking at the underlying motivations and background of the patient, but rather focusing on the interaction and the state of connectedness and resistance in the room.

An Analytic Attitude

All of the contributors advise us to try to assume a certain analytic attitude to better help and to tolerate masochistic patients and the pressures they place on us. Although they view origins differently, the techniques are designed to help the therapist/analyst maintain a respectfully empathic position most of the time and allow their understanding when they stray from the usual, even-hovering attention with analytic attitude. All would say that to remain empathic is difficult with sadomasochistic patients, but from a self-psychological framework, Ornstein's empathic mode refers to a means of listening and gathering the clinical data in the dyad.

Coen portrays the importance of the ability to tolerate hating and being hated while in the midst of sadomasochistic struggles in the transference/countertranference. He also describes how the analyst or therapist might utilize small emotional breaks in this containing attitude in order to avoid bigger breaks that destroy treatments. That is, to the degree that the therapist can catch and contain his interfering conflicts, he can then assist his patient to do so, too. He documented how such a break led to anger and higher resistance in the patient, whereas interpretation of the state of the patient's state of mind provided a positive link in the working alliance with the patient.

Other Technical Considerations

The authors share with us specific technical approaches and methods based on their experiences working with these difficult patients. These, of course, are linked to their understandings of the origins and meanings of the given masochistic phenomena.

Suicidal tendencies, self-harming symptoms and/or other high-risk behaviors can frequently accompany in various forms of masochistic patients and sometimes call for special interventions, such as confrontations about the dangerous behavior, the need for medication or hospitalization. The dyadic situation has to be made into a safe-enough setting, and a working relationship needs to be developed enough so that the suicidal sadomasochistic patient's acting-out can be optimally managed. At these times, the clinician will hope that the patient can accept "a gentle reality confrontation," as the Novicks put it. Moreover, many of the contributors advocate the importance of interpreting the conscious and unconscious meanings of such behaviors and the implications in the transference. For example, Ornstein elucidated the meanings of her patient's suicidal thoughts in terms of his deep anger at his maternal figures, his need for revenge and to show them to be "bad," his "feel sorry for me" attitude, and his deep sense of guilt. According to Margolis, a patient's suicidal threats can pull the therapist into being the rescuer and then can lead into significant boundary violations.

The Novicks offer a set of specific suggestions and approaches in dealing with "closed system" masochistic solutions patients may have and a set of specific suggestions and approaches in fostering "open system" approaches which would help these patients add to their defensive armamentarium.

Boundary Violations

All the authors illuminate sadomasochistic dynamics in the patient, but in Margolis's chapter we see how such dynamics and symptoms that become played out in the interactions between therapist and patient can lead to disaster in the treatment. Margolis demonstrates what can happen if the suggestions and warnings laid down by the other writers about recognizing, understanding, and utilizing sadomasochistic countertransferences go unheeded. Based on his experiences in ethics committees and in treating both violators and victims of sexual boundary violations, he explicates the intimate link between sadomasochistic problems in both patient and therapist when such boundary violations occur. In the typical scenarios outlined by Margolis, the clinician who is not able to tolerate the helpless feelings that are stirred up in working with sadomasochistic patients resorts to unconsciously omnipotent defenses. The therapist takes on the role of the rescuer which conceals the arrogant idea of "I can do anything." Narcissistic vulnerability closes off avenues for consultation with colleagues who could help in reality testing and leads to dysfunctional responses in which the therapist crosses boundaries and frequently commits sexual violations. He characterizes such violations "the tragic misalliances" that ruin careers and lives.

SUMMARY

We think that with these contributions, the clinical problem of masochism will no longer be a daunting uphill climb or an unsolvable mystery. They provide a series of sophisticated theoretical and clinical paradigms and guidelines for the treatment of sadomasochistic patients. For all the contributors, the patient's early environment plays a major etiologic role. All suggest that serious trauma, or cumulative trauma, is often part of the picture. All stress the importance of recognizing that masochistic symptoms and character are creative solutions to underlying problems. This recognition helps the clinician both to make sense of and to tolerate the patient's bewildering behavior and the difficult transferences and countertransferences that arise in the treatments. All argue and demonstrate clearly that the clinician must be able to understand and handle the inevitable countertransferences in order to bring about any significant change in these often entrenched symptoms and behaviors. While these authors demonstrate that we can work with most of the masochistic individuals most of the time, they also tell of the inevitable failures. They provide us with models for maintaining our equanimity with these difficult clinical situations and the knowledge that we are not alone in our difficult struggles. These authors present a framework in which to place, tolerate, and contain our own frustrations, pain, impotence, anger, and bewilderment.

REFERENCES

Brandchaft, B. (2007). Systems of pathological accommodations and change in analysis. *Psychoanalytic Psychology* 24: 667–87.

Coen, S. (1981). Sexualization as a predominant mode of defense. *Journal of the American Psychoanalytic Association* 29: 893–920.

——— (1992). *The Misuse of Persons: Analyzing Pathological Dependency.* Hillsdale, NJ: Analytic Press.

Cooper, A. M. (1988). The narcissistic-masochistic character. In *Masochism: Current Psychoanalytic Perspectives,* eds. R. A. Glick and D. I. Meyers. Hillsdale, NJ: Analytic Press, 117–38.

Cooper, A. M. (2009). The narcissistic-masochistic character. *Psychiatric Annals online.com* 39(10): 904–12.

Cooper, A. M., and Sacks, M. H. (1991). Sadism and masochism in character disorder and resistance. *Journal of the American Psychoanalytic Association* 39: 215–26.

Ellman, P. L. (2009). Battling the life and death forces of sadomasochism: Clinical perspectives from three cultures. Panel, Congress of International Psychoanalytical Association, Chicago, IL.

Freud, S. (1905). Three essays on sexuality. *Standard Edition* 7: 125–245.

——— (1919). A child is being beaten. *Standard Edition* 17: 175–204.

——— (1924). The economic problem of masochism. *Standard Edition* 19: 155–70.

——— (1937). Analysis terminable and interminable. *Standard Edition* 23: 209–53.

Gabbard, G. O. (2000). Hatred and its rewards: A discussion. *Psychoanalytic Inquiry* 20: 409–20.

Glick, R. A., and Meyers, D. I. (1988). Introduction. In *Masochism: Current Perspectives,* eds. R. A. Glick and D. I. Meyers. Hillsdale, NJ: Analytic Press, 1–25.

Goldberg, A. (1993). Sexualization and desexualization. *Psychoanalytic Quarterly* 62: 383–399.

Grotstein, J. M. (1984). A proposed revision of the psychoanalytic concept of primitive mental states, Part II—The borderline syndrome-Section 2 the phenomenology of the borderline syndrome. *Contemporary Psychoanalysis* 20: 77–19.

Horowitz, M. H. (1990). On beginning a reanalysis. In *On Beginning an Analysis,* eds. T. J. Jacobs and A. Rothstein. Madison, CT: International Universities Press, 101–13.

Joseph, B. (1982). Addiction to near-death. *International Journal of Psychoanalysis* 63: 449–56.

Kernberg, O. F. (1988). Clinical dimensions of masochism. *Journal of the American Psychoanalytic Association* 36: 1005–29.

——— (1991). Sadomasochism, sexual excitement, and perversion. *Journal of the American Psychoanalytic Association* 39: 333–62.

Novick, J., and Novick. K. K. (1987). The essence of masochism. *Psychoanalytic Study of the Child* 42: 353–84.

——— (1991). Some comments on masochism and the delusion of omnipotence from a developmental perspective. *Journal of the American Psychoanalytic Association* 39: 307–31.

ONE

Clinical Constellations of Masochistic Psychopathology

Otto F. Kernberg, MD

SOME GENERAL CONSIDERATIONS REGARDING MASOCHISM

One major problem in discussing masochistic psychopathology is the widening use of this concept within psychoanalysis and psychodynamic psychotherapy (Asch, 1988; Green, 2007). It raises the question, to what extent all forms of masochistic pathology warrant definition by two dominant psychodynamic constellations: 1) the need to suffer as a precondition for obtaining sexual pleasure, and 2) the dominance of severe superego pressures inducing guilt and the need of self-punishment for the unconscious implications of sexual and/or aggressive impulses. Related questions are whether the experience of pain in itself is an intrinsic aspect of sexual excitement—reflecting primary masochistic trends, and to what extent is it important to differentiate self-punishing behavior, intended to alleviate unconscious guilt, from self-destructive consequences of behavior, the original motivation for which is not related to unconscious guilt or superego pressures.

These conceptual issues affect how a broad spectrum of clinical constellations may be considered to be masochistic, and, in practice, throw light not only on different dynamic constellations, but on overall types of psychopathology that can be differentiated from each other, and have specific prognostic and therapeutic implications. In our clinical practice there seems to be no question that the severity of masochistic pathology differs widely between, say, on one extreme, patients who present with extreme self-mutilating behavior leading to the loss of limbs or self-castration, and the depressive-masochistic personality, a personality disorder at a neurotic level of organization, on the other.

From a psychoanalytic viewpoint, regarding the diagnostic evaluation of patients, an important question is to what extent the predominant unconscious dynamics determine prognosis, or, whether it is the degree to which the nature of the personality structure, regardless of the underlying dynamics, that determines the prognosis. In my view, to be reflected in what follows, it is the organization of the personality that determines analyzability and prognosis, while the unconscious individual dynamics, of course, will determine the course of the treatment, the nature and sequence of transference developments. Thus, for example, regarding masochistic perversion, analyzability and treatment in general depend on the underlying personality structure—that is, a masochistic perversion in a narcissistic personality structure has more negative prognostic implications than one in a patient with a hysterical personality. In this connection, one common practical problem is the frequent neglect of structural analysis of the patient's personality in the initial evaluation of patients, leading to potentially faulty indications or contraindications to psychoanalytic treatment (Kernberg, 1997).

The concept of primary masochism deserves a renewed interest. In the light of our present-day knowledge of the relation between neurobiological systems of affect activation and the effects of early object relations on the integration of affect dispositions, it appears that the combination of erotic excitement and pleasure in mildly painful bodily states may reflect an early condensation of sadistic and masochistic pleasure in identifying with the object of the sadistic approach (Kernberg, 2012a). The very early manifestation of the psychological features of this erotic and sadomasochistic combination may be seen in the tickling response, in the quality of teasing that emerges as such an essential aspect of sexual excitement and erotic attraction, and even the relief experienced by means of diffuse aggressive acts toward self and other, for example, lashing out, hitting and self-hitting, head banging, etc., may illustrate that combination of erotic excitement and active and passive painful experiences. Precursors of these aggressive aspects of erotic activation, on the one hand, and the pleasurable, diffuse lashing out at self and others, under the impact of intense aggressive affect activation, point to what used to be formulated as early fusion of aggressive and libidinal drives, and now may be reformulated as the effects of integration of peak affect states, both positive and negative, within the earliest object relations.

The work of Robert Stoller (1975, 1979, 1985) illustrated the importance of aggressive components of the erotic response in the polymorphous perverse features of sadistic, masochistic, voyeuristic, exhibitionistic, and fetishistic aspects of early eroticism. The somewhat addictive pleasurable relief in self-harming as part of the activation of intense negative affect storms of severe personality disorders, illustrates the counterpart, the heightening of self-directed as well as other directed aggression by a sense of erotic pleasure. From this perspective, polymorphous perverse infantile sexuality provides a major area for neutralization of aggression at the service of erotic strivings. Undifferentiated aggressive outbursts directed at one's own body, or someone else, provide a corresponding source of neutralization and relief from the intense pain of negative affect states.

From this normative recruitment of aggression at the service of eroticism, and the recruitment of an erotic response to reduce the intensity of pain related to negative affect activation, we may derive the conceptualization of masochistic pathology, in the most general terms, as the consolidation of major self-directed aggressive patterns in a defensive effort to control the diffuse, overwhelming, threatening effects of unbounded aggression, and the corresponding anxiety of fear of annihilation, elaborated along the parallel lines of consolidation of masochistic sexuality, on the one hand, and masochistic character formation, on the other. The basic origin of this pathology, both in the sexual and in the characterological realm, would be the internalization of real or fantasied, experienced or projected aggression in internalized self and object representations reflected in the earliest, sadistic level of superego precursors, and later, oedipally derived internalization of prohibitions and punishment against forbidden sexual as well as aggressive oedipal impulses in the definite superego structure (Kernberg, 1988, 2012b).

LEVELS OF MASOCHISTIC PATHOLOGY

From a developmental viewpoint, the various forms and degrees of severity of masochistic development might be formulated as a series of structures derived, respectively, from the developmental level of the psychic apparatus at which they develop and the degree to which aggressive realms of experience predominate over libidinal ones.

At the most extremely self-destructive level are the cases, mostly of psychotic patients, but including some borderline patients as well, whose severe self-mutilation and bodily self-destructiveness acquires deadly intensity. At the Personality Disorders Institute at Cornell, we have seen patients with a history of severe sexual abuse, specifically women who in their earliest childhood were violently sexually abused by alcoholic fathers, who later showed this syndrome of severely self-mutilating behavior in the context of borderline personality organization. One patient, raped by her alcoholic father at age ten, evinced self-mutilating behavior leading to the loss of fingers, paralysis of one arm, and an attempt at setting herself on fire that led to a major catastrophe affecting other inhabitants of her household. In short, at the most primitive level of self-directed aggression one observes the intent to erase all possibility of erotic activation, and self-aggression shows in unrelenting and severe self-mutilation in the context of borderline or even psychotic personality organization.

The next level of severity would be represented by the dominance of aggressive and self-aggressive behavior as a consequence of chronically traumatizing object relationships, such as is commonly reflected in the typical cases of borderline personality organization who present with practically total inhibition of all erotic sensual experience, absence of sexual arousal, no capacity for sexual excitement and orgasm even without self-mutilating behavior. Such cases present serious limitations in the prognosis for psychotherapeutic treatment, and are usually contraindicated for psychoanalysis proper. These patients frequently present minor self-cutting or other self-induced lesions, reporting that such behaviors reduce the intensity of intense affect and/or chronic tension. In the advanced stages of a specialized form of psychoanalytic psychotherapy, such as Transference Focused Psychotherapy, having achieved significant improvement of their capacity for more mature object relations, these patients may develop intense fantasies of a primitive sadomasochistic sexual nature, fantastic scenarios of polymorphous perverse infantile features, with overwhelming predominance of sadomasochistic features that may be resolved only slowly in the transference analysis of their repetition of earliest traumatic experiences. The heretofore pervasive elimination of erotic and dependent internalized object relations by the predominance of primitive aggression reaches a dramatic intensity in their transference developments.

At a higher level of borderline personality organization, with somewhat less severe dominance of self-destructiveness, the usual splitting between idealized and persecutory segments of experience may be dominant, and polymorphous perverse infantile sexual behavior emerges in the form of multiple, contradictory, perverse features of sexual excitement without the specific consolidation of a perversion proper in the sense of a specific masochistic precondition for achieving sexual excitement and orgasm. Here, masochistic sexual trends represent, paradoxically, precursors of a more normal recruitment of sadomasochistic features at the service of sexual excitement and eroticism, even if these features are significantly exaggerated in an effort to deal with the consequences of severe physical or sexual traumatization. Characterologically, in these patients, chaotic relationships with clinging dependency as well as aggressive distancing may include unstable sadomasochistic patterns of interpersonal interaction. But, in all these cases, we see no clinical evidence of consolidated superego functions and very little evidence of unconscious guilt as codeterminator of masochistic sexual behavior or self-defeating characterological behavior. Efforts to control overwhelming aggression may be channeled, alternatively, into sadomasochistic behavior patterns or accentuation of the aggressive components of polymorphous infantile sexuality, and the constellation of primitive defensive operations related to splitting mechanism dominate psychic structure, as well as behavior patterns. At this level of pathology, one sees few patients with a consolidated, stable sexual perversion: such a stable perversion usually would indicate a higher level of superego integration, and a reduced dominance of splitting operations. Here the dynamics of the perversion, derived from oedipal and pre-oedipal levels of development, overlap strikingly with the unconscious dynamics of borderline personality organization in general (Chasseguet-Smirgel, 1984; Kernberg 1992; Lussier, 1983; Stoller, 1975).

In any case, patients with borderline personality organization and chaotic polymorphous perverse infantile sexual behavior represent a higher level of development, and better prognosis for treatment than those in which overwhelming primitive aggression has eliminated the possibility for sensual erotic experience, as well as determining the most primitive self-destructive characterological features.

The consolidation of a pathological grandiose self in narcissistic personality organization represents a further development of the defensive structures directed against primitive aggression and a consolidated sexual perversion may be crystalized in the context of such a personality structure. On the other hand, when aggression, both self and other directed, is expressed mostly in the patient's character constellation, we find the "thin skinned" narcissistic patients (Rosenfeld, 1987), who present both severe infiltration of the pathological grandiose self with aggression, and a structural weakness of the pathological grandiose self, so that shifts from states of arrogance, superiority and contemptuous feelings about the analyst evolve in alternation with severe feelings of inferiority, humiliation, depression, self-accusation and suicidal tendencies. Their clinical presentation may include intense characterological depression or chronic dysthymic reactions, suicidal tendencies, marked experiences of emptiness, uncertainty and confusion about one's life and relations, and ego syntonic sadistic features, both expressed and projected onto the analyst. In these cases severe, dangerous, suicidal self-destructiveness may express unconscious fantasies of superiority by defying the usual human fears over pain, illness or death, and represent an unconscious triumph over those who try to help them. Severe cases of masochistic-narcissistic personalities also correspond to this primitive level of masochistic pathology (Cooper, 1989).

Masochistic perversions in the context of these narcissistic personality structures may be characterized by extreme, even life-threatening sexual behaviors and submission to a humiliating control in the context of an absence of any emotional relationship and any stable, self-contained boundaries of such a perversion: the perverse behavior fits into the context of a lack of significant object relationships and is usually interspersed with severe sadistic tendencies. At this level of masochistic pathology, however, from a dynamic viewpoint, one finds the complex combination of pre-oedipal and oedipal conflicts under the predominance of pre-oedipal aggression that characterizes all perversions at the borderline level.

In contrast, at a next higher level of development, with a normal integration of the tripartite psychic structure, sexual perversions correspond to the classical Freudian model that implies the expression of profound unconscious guilt over the incestuous and parricidal implications of sexuality that underlie specific sexual perversions, including sexual masochism (Kernberg, 1997). Here we find specific unconscious sexual scenarios embedded within the context of a capacity for deep and potentially even mature object relations, with the characteristic features of the masochistic scenarios, that is, the requirement of pain, of being controlled, and of being humiliated as an indispensable precondition for achievement of sexual excitement and orgasm. If unconscious superego "absorbed" aggression can be gratified by this sexual restriction, and the secondary idealization of this perversion as an ideal sexual relationship can be sustained, the denial of castration anxiety may be assured. Here we no longer see the more primitive dynamics described by Chasseguet-Smirgel (1984) of perversion at the borderline level, in which an unconscious denial of the difference between genders and generations, and of oedipal rivalry is achieved in the unconscious elimination of all boundaries to sexual engagements. At the level of neurotic personality organization, in contrast, the combination of the enjoyment of pain, suffering and humiliation becomes the direct expression of a superego determined compromise formation that protects sexual intimacy within the restriction of a perversion.

Also, at the level of neurotic personality organization, masochistic tendencies may be expressed preferentially through characterological patterns, specifically the depressive-masochistic personality disorder (Kernberg, 1988). Such patients are characterized by pathological patterns reflecting unconscious superego pressure: excessive seriousness, somberness, a bleak experience of life, a restricted sense of humor, and over-conscientiousness, a high level of dependability and responsibility combined with hard self-judgments and self-devaluation (if one does not live up to one's high moral standards and demands for work). The relationship between unconscious feelings of guilt over oedipal rivalry, and oedipal sexuality in general, is indirectly expressed in these behavioral patterns, as well as in regressive dependent features. These patients are notable for excessive dependency and easy frustratibility, vulnerability to feeling let down and disappointed, a tendency to self-sacrifice and excessive compliance to others in order to receive love, while, at the same time, they also may unconsciously try to control others through generating guilt feelings in them. Sometimes an excessive self-reliance or independence constitutes a reaction formation against excessive dependent needs, but when their dependent needs are frustrated, they tend to develop depressive reactions.

In general, these patients show what may be considered a faulty metabolism of aggression, reflecting excessive superego prohibitions against anger and rage: they get depressed under conditions when it would be reasonable for them to get angry; there is an excessive fear of being criticized for self-affirmative behavior, and they may combine a harsh, critical tendency toward others in unconscious identification with their own superego demands, with yet excessive guilt over these attacks on others. Again, while their conflicts around dependency indicate the regression and or participation of pre-oedipal issues in their dominant oedipal conflicts, there is a clear dominance of these latter themes in their unconscious conflicts, in the context of a general high level of functioning, normal identity formation, and the related capacity for object relationships in depth.

The depressive-masochistic personality disorder, however, may evince regressive characterological features that indicate the intensity of aggressive dispositions that emerge in combination with splitting mechanisms, and show clinically in sadomasochistic character features, in which all the previously mentioned masochistic features are combined, with the tendency of unconscious sadism expressed in their excessive criticism and efforts to control others. Here the unconscious efforts to control others through the induction of feelings of guilt may become a dominant characterological feature.

Both the disturbances in the sexual life of patients with a masochistic perversion and their dominant masochistic characterological patterns significantly influence these patients' love life. The nature of the conflicts in their love life, in fact, is strongly determined by the predominant nature of their personality organization, that is, the extent to which borderline personality organization, a narcissistic personality disorder, or neurotic personality organization are the context in which masochistic sexual behavior and/or characterological patterns emerge. The general chaos of interpersonal relationships, the combination of clinging dependency and aggressive reactions in the context of chaotic love relations is characteristic of borderline patients. Here, however, in the middle of such chaos, patients still may have the capacity to fall in love, to establish deep and dependent, even if clinging, relationships, and evince a greater potential for stability of love relations than narcissistic patients, whose surface functioning frequently seems to be much better.

Narcissistic patients' incapacity to fall in love, the presence of transitory infatuations and repeated devaluation of the love objects determines narcissistic forms of sexual promiscuity, distinguishable from masochistic sexual promiscuity in which potentially gratifying love relations are undermined and destroyed, with the patient only settling into a stable, but clearly masochistic relationship, often with a narcissistic or sadistic love object. A frequent history of disappointing love relations is typical for masochistic personalities, and also shows in their selection of unavailable or potentially frustrating objects—that is, the typical longing of masochistic patients for narcissistic partners. Unconscious collusions of couples who, au fond, have a happy relationship which generates inordinate guilt and a mutual collusion to create some destructive features in their relationship as a price to pay for its survival, are perhaps as frequent as the breakdowns of the relationships of couples with one or both severely narcissistic partners.

A final issue to be considered is the sublimatory potential of the universality of masochistic dispositions. Masochistic pathology, as has been stressed, is a consequence of the dominance of aggressive strivings that are "metabolized" at various levels of psychological development within the respectively dominant personality organization, into the patient's sexual life, the patient's character structure, or both. Yet, as André Green (2007) has pointed out, self-destructive tendencies, unconscious temptations toward self-defeating, self-undermining behaviors are probably universal, and reflect the ever present potential for regression in superego functions. By the same token, however, the sublimatory role of self-sacrifice in the service of a major ideal may reflect a mature emotional disposition that implies a creative potential. Hard work and suffering at the service of creativity and art or science, in effectiveness and productivity, reflect such utilization of suffering in the service of an ego syntonic goal. That function may be corrupted by superego pathology into a self-destructive commitment to anti-humanistic goals, such as, for example, the severe sadomasochistic aspects of politically rationalized violence and terrorism, or, in more subtle sadistic expression of the tyrannical suppression of others at the service of one's own pseudo-idealistic goals. With the mature development of internalized value systems, a spirit of responsible commitment to social goals and self-sacrifice may fulfill personal sublimatory functions as well as community goals. In any case, a concerned alertness to self-defeating, self-destructive tendencies that may be activated in decision making processes under conditions of uncertainty is one of the mature psychological functions of decision making.

By the same token, the sublimatory recruitment of sadistic and masochistic impulses at the service of erotic excitement is an important source of enrichment of erotic phantasy, play, and interaction, frequently inhibited by superego pressures generated in the love life of a couple, that needs to be diagnosed and, at times, freed from repression.

DIAGNOSTIC AND THERAPEUTIC CONSIDERATIONS

In the diagnostic evaluation of patients with masochistic character pathology, it is important to evaluate to what extent, what they consider their "normal" life situation, their work, love relations, social environment, family relations, their conformity with these life circumstances may, by itself, disguise significant masochistic features, in terms of aspirations denied, talents neglected, problematic life situations that could be changed, accepted as normal. There are cultural conventionalities that may influence both the patient's and the analyst's judgment: unhappy love affairs, in my experience, tend to be more frequently diagnosed as reflecting significant masochistic features when they are experienced by women, but not men; while pathological submission to frustrating, destructive or demeaning work situations evinced by men may frequently be ignored because of a conventional ideology that expects men to remain in tough work conditions. Similarly, women who sacrifice their professional knowledge and talents under the rationalization of full dedication to their children and families may also fit traditional social expectations, allowing their masochistic features to be missed. It may appear banal to stress the importance of carefully evaluating a couple's sexual life in terms of their emotional relationship, their value systems, and their sexual fantasy, play, and behavior. Unfortunately, many psychotherapists, including psychoanalysts, neglect a full evaluation of sexual life in the initial diagnostic study of patients and tend to miss masochistic restrictions to their mutual pleasure producing interactions.

Finally, there are important general aspects to the diagnostic evaluation that have fundamental importance in establishing a prognostic estimate: above all, the predominant personality structure of the patient, in addition to the severity of self-directed aggression, the depth and maturity of object relations, and the extent of mature, in contrast to infantile, rigid, or defective, superego integration.

Regarding therapeutic considerations, the vast field of masochistic pathology within the broad context outlined in this presentation defies simple generalizations. Severe depressive-masochistic personality disorders, chronic masochistic behavior in the context of a couple's love relationship, and a masochistic perversion at a level of neurotic personality organization warrant psychoanalytic treatment and present an overall favorable prognosis. A major problem in the transference developments, in these cases, is the activation of superego derived aggression in the transference, when the patient unconsciously attempts to fight off the analyst's efforts to help him/her, persisting in self-defeating behavior as part of an unconscious identification with internalized sadistic objects. The analysis of this particular enacted object relationship between superego and ego structures may contribute fundamentally to resolving the unconscious masochistic pressures. In the case of masochistic perversion at a neurotic level, the exploration and working through of the highly individualized unconscious psychodynamics of the perverse scenarios in the transference situation appears an essential precondition for the resolution of such a perversion, a general principle valid for the treatment of all crystalized perversions at a neurotic level.

Under the condition of sexual masochism or severely sadomasochistic character patterns in the context of a narcissistic personality disorder, the systematic working through and resolution of the activation of the pathological grandiose self in the transference, its gradual decomposition in the component ideal self and ideal object representations and the sadistic components of these internalizations require patient and long-term transference analysis, with the analyst prepared to deal with temporary, severe regression into more primitive paranoid and sadomasochistic transferences. The most severe cases are represented by patients with borderline personality organization, with diffuse and pervasive self-destructiveness as part of a general expression of primitive aggressive behaviors toward others and self, with relatively limited superego functions involved, and a clear dominance of splitting operations and related primitive defenses: here a modification of psychoanalytic technique, the utilization of specialized psychoanalytic psychotherapies such as transference focused psychotherapy for borderline conditions may replace the indications for analysis proper (Clarkin, Yeomans, and Kernberg, 2006). The treatment of these patients requires setting up of clear treatment boundaries and limits that protect the patient, the therapist, and potentially others from severe acting out of self-destructive and/or sadistic tendencies. This, particularly, is relevant for patients with chronic, severe, non-depressive suicidal behavior and a history of frequent hospitalizations related to suicidal attempts in the past. Our advances in the psychoanalytic psychotherapy for these cases have effectively broadened the field of treatment for most severe masochistic pathology, although there still remain cases where the unconscious motivation to self-destruct reflects what might be called, practically, clinical manifestations of the death drive, and treatment may become almost impossible, particularly if the indispensable structural arrangements to protect the patient and the treatment cannot be established and maintained. Patients who engage in repeated suicidal and parasuicidal behavior that gravely threatens their survival, and who manifest antisocial and litigious behavior that threatens the therapist, illustrate this area of pathology. Our technical knowledge and possibilities have significantly advanced, it seems to me, over the past twenty years to a state where the large majority of patients with masochistic pathology may now be treated with psychoanalysis and derived techniques, but our best efforts, and most experienced therapists cannot prevent that some patients will not survive their self-destructive urges.

There are some technical principles regarding the management of masochistic transferences that apply across the entire spectrum of masochistic pathology. One such understanding is that, in the case of sexual masochism, as in all cases of sexual perversion, psychoanalytic resolution of this pathology requires the systematic and in-depth exploration of the masochistic scenario in the transference. The analytic work of exploring the unconscious meaning of the sexual scene involves the activation of the corresponding object relations in their sexual interactions, and powerful resistances may operate against the full deployment of them in the transference. The patient's sexual engagements may increasingly serve the purpose of acting out the transference, and because the masochistic sexual behavior predates the analysis, this changing function of the masochistic symptom may be recognized only slowly by the analyst.

In the case of characterological masochistic pathology, ("moral masochism"), patients may not only chronically project their persecutory superego onto the analyst, but alternatate between periods where they feel attacked and devalued by the analyst, and other periods where, in identification with the persecutory superego, their own sadistic behavior and devaluation of the analyst dominate. And in still other periods of the treatment, the patients' self-accusations and self-attacks signal the intrapsychic expression of the masochistic pathology, the simultaneous identification with victim and persecutor, with an implicit dismissal of the analyst's interventions reflecting the acting out of unconscious guilt. In the cases with narcissistic pathology, in turn, that dismissal of the analyst's interventions may express the self-destructive grandiosity of the pathological grandiose self, typical for the masochistic-narcissistic personalities described by Cooper (1989).

One other significant complication is the development of negative therapeutic reactions reflecting unconscious guilt, typical for depressive masochistic personality structures. Originally described by Freud (1920, 1924), negative therapeutic reaction as an expression of unconscious guilt represents a regressive superego defense against the sense of being helped and freed from excessive superego pressures. While negative therapeutic reaction derived from unconscious envy of the analyst in narcissistic personality structure is, by far, more frequent, masochistic pathology often goes hand in hand with a propensity to negative therapeutic reactions that sometimes emerges in late stages of the treatment and needs to be interpreted consistently.

Another important complication within the most severe types of masochistic pathology is the development of severe suicidal tendencies reflecting the character pathology and not actual depressive reactions, leading therapists to treating assumed major depressions with medication, rather than analyzing the unconscious meaning of these characterological defenses as transference resistances. These developments may be observed in patients with depressive-masochistic character structure, but particularly in patients with borderline personality organization, and with severe narcissistic pathology. The presence of strong suicidal trends in borderline patients without depression represents an indication for high priority interpretation of the unconscious meanings of their suicidal impulses in the transference, combined with a clear structure of the treatment that commits the patient to either discuss suicidal tendencies in the sessions or, if the patient senses that he cannot control his behavior, by consulting a psychiatric emergency room. The interpretation of the transference implications of such limit setting becomes part of the interpretation of the unconscious meanings of the suicidal ideation and intention at that point. This is an area within which Transference Focused Psychotherapy has developed effective modifications of psychoanalytic technique for borderline personality organization, and where standard psychoanalytic technique needs to incorporate the technical interventions stemming from the experience of psychoanalytic psychotherapy with severe personality disorders (Clarkin et al., 2006).

Finally, frequent countertransference reactions to patients with masochistic character pathology deserve to be mentioned. These patients, often having ruined important opportunities for success and happiness in their lives, may elicit a sense of pity and commiseration by the therapist, particularly if they manage to convincingly present their sense of hopelessness of their situation. Pity reflects a submission to the patient's superego, and it may also be a reaction formation against a therapist's resentment of the patient's unconscious efforts to project guilt feelings onto him. The opposite reaction, resentment and an internal giving up on a patient who systematically undermines all efforts by the analyst to help through understanding, may lead to impulsive disruption or termination of the treatment. Obviously, the analyst or therapist needs to tolerate his/her aggression in the countertransference, and utilize it in the formulation of transference interpretations without having to deny, act out, or share these feelings with the patient. An appropriate therapeutic distance usually will permit, without too much difficulty, to sort out the patient's self-defeating maneuvers from what, at first sight, may appear an extremely realistic, bad life situation. If the therapist, faced with what seems a patient's impossible life situation, can envision internally a way to confront it effectively if the therapist himself/herself were in that predicament, the patient's prognosis improves by that very fact.

REFERENCES

Asch, S. S. (1988). The analytic concepts of masochism: A reevaluation. In *Masochism: Current Psychoanalytic Perspectives*, eds. R. A. Glick and D. J. Meyers. Hillsdale, NJ: Analytic Press, 93–115.

Chasseguet-Smirgel, J. (1984). *Creativity and Perversion*. New York: W. W. Norton.

Clarkin, J. F., Yeomans, F. E., and Kernberg, O. F. (2006). *Psychotherapy for Borderline Personality: Focusing on Object Relations*. Washington, D.C.: American Psychiatric Publishing.

Cooper, A. M. (1989). Narcissism and masochism: The narcissistic-masochistic character. *Psychiatric Clinics of North America* 12(3): 541–52.

Freud, S. (1920). Beyond the pleasure principle. *Standard Edition* 18: 1–64.

—— (1924). The economic problem of masochism. *Standard Edition* 19: 155–70.

Green, A. (2007). The death drive: Meaning, objections, substitutes. In *Reading French Psychoanalysis*, eds. D. Birksted-Breen, S. Flanders, and A. Gibeault. London: Routledge, 2010, 496–515.

Kernberg, O. F. (1988). Clinical dimensions of masochism. In *Masochism: Current Psychoanalytic Perspectives*, eds. R. A. Glick and D. J. Meyers. Hillsdale, NJ: Analytic Press, 61–79.

—— (1992). *Aggression in Personality Disorders and Perversion*. New Haven: Yale University Press, 245–92.

—— (1997). Perversion, perversity, and normality: Diagnostic and therapeutic considerations. *Psychoanalysis and Psychotherapy* 14: 19–40.

—— (2012a) The sexual couple: A psychoanalytic exploration. In *The Inseparable Nature of Love and Aggression*. Washington, D.C.: American Psychiatric Publishing, 247–72.

—— (2012b). Sexual Pathology in Borderline Patients. In *The Inseparable Nature of Love and Aggression*. Washington, D.C.: American Psychiatric Publishing, 293–306.

Lussier, A. (1983). Les deviations du dèsir. Etude sur le fetichisme. *Revue Française de Psychoanalyse* 47: 19–142.

Rosenfeld, H. (1987). *Impasse and Interpretation*. London: Routledge, 274.

Stoller, R. (1975). *Perversion: The Erotic Form of Hatred*. Washington, D.C.: American Psychiatric Press.

—— (1979). *Sexual Excitement*. New York: Pantheon.

—— (1985). *Observing the Erotic Imagination*. New Haven: Yale University Press.

TWO

Masochism in Childhood and Adolescence as a Self-Regulatory Disorder

Alan Sugarman, PhD

Twenty years ago I published an article about a three-year-old girl who suffered from prominent masochistic pathology (Sugarman, 1991a) and marked beating fantasies (Sugarman, in press) that colored her entire analysis. The vivid nature of her masochism, its origins in cumulative trauma, as well its underlying dynamic and structural contributors, all proved useful in clarifying various aspects of child psychoanalytic technique with such psychopathology including the use of play (Sugarman, 2008) and the nature of such a child's termination phase (Sugarman, 1991b). In other words, this little girl's difficulties and the way she expressed and analyzed them proved a virtual treasure trove of psychoanalytic data. Yet, despite her masochism being so interesting and illuminating as to inspire four scholarly publications, I was not allowed to call her masochistic in the original paper. Instead the reviewers and editor mandated that I adhere to standard analytic practice at that time and refer to her pathology as proto-masochistic because she was too young to have her symptoms rooted in oedipal conflicts (e.g., Galenson, 1988; Glenn, 1989). Thus, I was required to state: "In general, it is the traversal of the oedipal stage and the compromise formations arising from it that determine ultimately whether or not there will be a masochistic resolution and what form it will take. Consequently, those pre-oedipal conflicts or forerunners of later masochistic phenomena tend to be considered 'protomasochistic'" (Sugarman, 1991a, p. 107).

But the clinical experience and confidence that I have gained over the past two decades since first writing about Sarah lead me to believe that it is time to reconsider these distinctions. Since that time, I have analyzed children as young as two and a half with significant masochistic pathology that appears no different in structure or dynamics than masochistic pathology in older children and adults except for the absence of oedipal contributors. Such experience suggests that the main reason for continuing to distinguish between masochistic and protomasochistic pathology is our discipline's collective tendency to adhere to traditional theoretical concepts and technical principles that originated with Freud. One of these shibboleths is the prioritizing of the Oedipus complex in understanding psychopathology. Despite the empirically documented findings of the Novicks (Novick and Novick, 1987) that every developmental stage contributes to the formation of masochistic symptoms or character traits, we continue to write and theorize as though the oedipal stage with its characteristic triangular conflict is the most important stage and conflict for elucidating etiology.

Freud's classic paper, "A Child is Being Beaten" (1919), essentially explained such masochistic fantasies as due to unconscious guilt over oedipal longings leading to their repression and expression in fantasy only (Glick and Meyers, 1988). And even these fantasies were often repressed, becoming conscious only during analysis. This emphasis on unconscious guilt in masochism was so important, along with its other manifestation in negative therapeutic reactions, that it was a major impetus to Freud replacing the topographic model with the structural one some four years later. But even after introducing the structural model in 1923 in "The Ego and the Id," Freud maintained his oedipal prioritization in explaining masochism. It remained central in "The Economic Problem of Masochism" (Freud, 1924) one year after his theoretical revision. "Turning his attention to the clinical manifestations of masochism, which could now be explained by his instinct theory, Freud again grounded the vicissitudes and the consequent structure of the mental apparatus firmly in the instincts" (Glick and Meyers, 1988, p. 7).

Yet such a formulation, if it is accepted, would require us to call masochistic pathology in children younger than six years old something else, most commonly protomasochistic. And this is often the case despite questions being raised about Freud's minimization of pre-oedipal stages and conflicts for at least half a century. Bergler (1961), for example, dated masochism to the first eighteen months of life. Similarly, Valenstein (1973) traced it to separation-individuation experiences and conflicts while Burgner and Kennedy (1980) noted the prominence of anal stage issues. And many analysts over the years have challenged Freud's singleminded emphasis on oedipal contributors to the beating fantasy and his finding/assumption that the beater is always the father in the fantasy (Asch, 1980; Bergler, 1948; Ferber and Gray, 1966; Galenson, 1980; Lester,

1957; Modell, 1997; Myers, 1980; Novick and Novick, 1972; Rubenfine, 1965; Schmideberg, 1948; Shengold, 1997). Hence, clinical experience has led many away from blind allegiance to outdated ideas in a way that can allow for broader recognition of the pervasiveness of masochistic pathology in children, even quite young ones, as well as to a reconsideration of just what are the dynamic, structural and perhaps environmental precipitants of such pathology.

The next section of this chapter will examine more carefully some of the pathogenic issues and questions that have been obscured by the common tendency to assume that masochism is grounded in the Oedipus complex. I will not spend time exploring the complexity of how to define masochism. That is a subject worthy of a paper in its own right and there are already many excellent ones in the literature (e.g., Grossman, 1986; Maleson, 1984; Novick and Novick, 1996). For the purposes of this chapter, any symptoms, behavior or personality traits in which a child consciously or unconsciously links pleasure and unpleasure in a motivated and automatic way will be considered masochistically pathological. That is, these manifestations will indicate that the child cannot experience important pleasures without causing pain to be inflicted on himself or herself. It is this obligatory linking of pleasure and pain that differentiates masochistic phenomena from other neurotic ones that have more general, and not necessarily intentional, self-defeating aspects.

WHY HAS THE OEDIPUS COMPLEX BEEN
SEEN AS SO IMPORTANT?

As mentioned above, the Oedipus complex has been the benchmark for differentiating neuroses from other more serious types of psychopathology since Freud (Fenichel, 1945). Thus, psychoanalysts training through the 1980s were taught to formulate their neurotic patients' psychopathology as rooted in oedipal conflicts and fantasies or traumas from that developmental stage. Such grounding became particularly important because psychoanalysis proper was thought to be the treatment of choice for neurotic patients. Generations of analysts were forced to plow their way through Fenichel's tome (1945) with its arcane and heavily metapsychological language in order to defend such treatment recommendations. Were one not able to make a case that his or her patient's psychopathology was rooted in oedipal conflicts, one would have to conclude that the patient was narcissistic or borderline and needed to be treated with *only* psychotherapy or parameters. Patients with conflicts in which dependent or narcissistic wishes predominated, or ones who were clearly conflicted around separation-individuation strivings, had to be considered "pre-oedipal" and, therefore, not the ideal patient for psychoanalysis. Given the importance of oedipal roots, child and adult patients were subjected to strained diagnostic formulations in which such pre-oedipal mental content, or others of similar ilk, were said to involve defensive regressions from oedipal conflicts that were simply too anxiety or guilt provoking to remain at that level. In this way, diagnostic formulations began to involve an infinite regress in which any sort of symptom, character trait, dynamic, etc. could be said to involve such a defensive regression (Brown and Sugarman, 2002). Diagnostic thinking became so strained and convoluted that the term neurosis virtually disappeared from the analytic literature in the last two decades (Sugarman, 2007). The diagnostic category of masochism became one of the many casualties of our discipline's unwillingness to reconsider its model of pathogenesis.

Only in the last fifteen years have a few psychoanalysts suggested the need to disentangle the psychodynamic, oedipal conflict from the degree and kinds of mental structure that come together and coalesce during the ages of four to six, the years usually referred to as the oedipal stage of development. Tyson (1996a, 1996b) has been one of the most articulate. Her major point is that it is certain structural accomplishments during the oedipal stage of development, not the instinctual conflict that occurs during it, that differentiate a neurotically organized mind from a non-neurotically organized one. This emphasis on the diagnostic importance of mental structure, and de-emphasis on drive vicissitudes, is yet another corrective to the "developmental lag" noted by Gray (1994) and Busch (1995) in integrating the clinical implications of the structural model into our everyday ways of understanding and working with patients.

This subtle but important shift in diagnostic criteria has important repercussions for the traditional distinction between masochism and protomasochism. In essence, it suggests that the level of drive conflict is not a relevant distinction. As the Novicks (Novick and Novick, 1996) have found, all levels of drive development that have been engaged will contribute to and be represented in masochistic symptoms or character traits. What is truly relevant is the degree and nature of the mental structure contributing to these phenomena. The automatic and obligatory linking of pleasure and unpleasure mentioned above implies a degree of intentionality, albeit usually unconscious. And such intentionality requires a modicum of mental structure for it to occur. Complex unconscious intentionality cannot happen in a mind that has not achieved some cognitive development, defensive capacities, representational boundaries, etc. It seems that a more legitimate way to determine if certain symptoms or character traits are masochistic would be to clarify if they exist in a mind that has the requisite structure to be capable of such intentional linking of pleasure and unpleasure. If so, there would seem to be no useful purpose in distinguishing between masochism proper and protomasochism. Toward this end, the next section will consider some of the key structural features of masochism emphasized in the literature.

STRUCTURAL FEATURES OF MASOCHISM

The Superego

The superego has been linked to masochism since the formulations of unconscious guilt giving rise to beating fantasies. It is impossible to explain the affect of guilt without a superego concept. And traditional thought has always linked the development of the superego to resolution of the Oedipus complex. "Freud proposed that the superego results from crucial identifications made with the father during efforts to avoid feared castration and to resolve oedipal conflicts (1923, pp. 28–39). It is therefore formed upon oedipal resolution, which is why he described the superego as the 'heir of the Oedipus complex'" (Tyson and Tyson, 1990, p. 199). One continues to see and hear this formulation in the literature, clinical discussions and analytic classrooms. For example, "Normal latency begins as the Oedipal child increasingly aware that he or she cannot win the dangerous conflict, gradually replaces the desire to challenge the parent of the same sex with the wish to be like him or her. The transition is facilitated by the formation of a new psychic structure—the superego" (Colarusso, 1992, p. 79). This obligatory linking of superego functioning with oedipal resolution continues to occur despite the challenges of many like Holder (1982) who argues that the relationship between these is often overstated.

If Holder and others (Tyson and Tyson, 1990) are correct that superego development is not so inextricably tied to instinctual development, particularly the Oedipus complex, the assumption that oedipal resolution is necessary to characterize phenomena as masochistic is certainly open to challenge. And both developmental data (Tyson and Tyson, 1984) as well as clinical evidence (Sugarman, 1999) indicate far earlier superego formation and functioning. One has only to examine the case of Bobby (Sugarman, 1999; 2003a) to find masochistic symptoms related to a punitive and functioning superego in an anal stage child. Bobby was two and one half when his parents consulted me about his extreme regression following ear tube surgery several months earlier. Despite thoughtful and excellent preparation for the surgery, Bobby's behavior changed markedly after it; he became unusually oppositional, angry and defiant and lost the urinary and bowel control he had attained for some months before the surgery. He attacked his parents and older brother physically, threw things at glass doors and windows in defiance of parental prohibition, grabbed toys from friends while accusing them of being "bad" and became dangerously wild, courting disaster by running into streets, climbing to dangerous heights, etc. Encopretic symptoms went beyond the norm as he deposited his stools on his father's desk and mother's sewing chair. In summary, he seemed completely out of control. Behavioral interventions proved of no use, leading his father's analyst to refer the parents to me.

Space constraints prevent a detailed description of his analysis. Suffice it to say, the analytic material provided ample evidence that superego conflicts played a prominent role in the genesis and maintenance of his symptoms. Essentially, his symptoms represented a regressive response to his superego attacks, and an attempt to elicit punishment, both to regulate guilt over aggressive impulses and to forestall even greater danger from harsh superego criticism. They also involved an attempt to attach masochistically to critical and poorly attuned parents. Hence, his seemingly impulsive and poorly regulated behavior proved to reflect intense intrapsychic conflict in which punitive superego injunctions against aggressive impulses played a significant role. His material ultimately revealed that he had interpreted the precipitating surgery as a punishment for his "badness" by which he meant his aggressive (not yet oedipal) impulses. Thus, I concluded:

> The prominence of Bobby's superego in the etiology of his encopresis highlights the coherence and influence of the superego far earlier than oedipal resolution. The degree to which it participated in his symptom picture seems to warrant it being considered more than a superego precursor. . . . When a superego exerts as prominent and consistent an impact on a child's inner world as Bobby's did, it seems unnecessary and even inconsistent with the clinical data to call it a precursor and differentiate it from the superego proper only because its content is preoedipal. (Sugarman, 1999, p. 514)

That is, the distinction between superego precursors and a mature superego suggested by some (Tyson and Tyson, 1984) can seem artificial when looking at actual analytic data. This young boy's superego seemed functionally no different than a latency aged superego (see Sugarman, 1994). To be sure, its primitive criticalness caused him to turn to masochistic provocativeness in order to regulate it. But such criticalness is no different than one sees in older children and adults with a variety of neurotic symptoms. Thus, there appears to be no reason for calling his symptoms protomasochistic instead of masochistic.

The Representational World

Asch (1976) has also contributed to expanding the diagnostic criteria for masochism earlier than the oedipal stage with his work on the negative therapeutic reaction, one of the most common analytic manifestations of masochism. In contrast to Freud's emphasis on unconscious guilt stemming from a critical and punitive superego, Asch notes pathology of the ego ideal as seen in trying to appease or identifying with a sadistic or masochistic parental introject. For example, the masochistic patient's pursuit of suffering can: "reflect libidinal strivings toward the internalized object in the ego ideal, epitomized by the suffering martyr. As a result, the dominant aim of their object relations is masochistic, the dominant object remains internalized in the ego ideal" (p. 386). At other times the masochistic patient is searching for love from an introject who is sadistic rather than loving (Asch, 1976; Berliner, 1947). Obeying these introjects both alleviates guilt and brings the narcissistic gratification of gaining the introject's approval. In this way suffering and pleasure become linked in an attempt to regulate self-esteem.

But the internalization of introjects and efforts to please them occur far earlier than the oedipal stage, let alone resolution of the Oedipus complex. Remorse, shame, and guilt when not pleasing these introjects are reported to occur as early as two-and-one-half years old (Tyson and Tyson, 1990). And a "loveable" self image occurs when the toddler feels that he or she has, indeed, pleased the introject (R. L. Tyson, 1983). One could observe these reactions in Bobby, discussed above. Furthermore, Bobby's parents' attitudes toward and interactions with him created the sort of representational world that inevitably leads to masochism. This should not be surprising because pain seeking symptomatolgy has been linked to disturbed early mother-child relationships (Glenn, 1984a, 1984b, 1989; Novick and Novick, 1996; Valenstein, 1973). An inability to soothe the infant for whatever the reason interferes with the internalization and formation of a pleasurable and comforting representational world. Instead, masochistic patients are often "individuals whose attachment to pain signifies an original attachment to perceived objects" (Valenstein, 1973, p. 389). Bobby's parents perceived him as more active, and hence difficult, from the time he was still a fetus in utero. His early months were characterized by intense gastro-intestinal pain that was more pervasive and early than typical colic. Hence his mother could not soothe him. Eventually, she noticed that not eating spicy foods alleviated his symptoms. But he would have associated his early mothering with pain by that time. Furthermore, his parents' not verbalized but clearly expressed disapproval of his temperament and activity level required him to attach to objects that caused subtle, narcissistic pain in every interaction with him. Masochism became his way to regulate the pain and fear of object loss or loss of his parents' love.

There is significant consensus among modern analysts of various theoretical persuasions that other qualities and vicissitudes of early internalized self and object representations also play a major causal role in masochism (Asch, 1988; Glick and Meyers, 1988; Kernberg, 1988; Sarnoff, 1988). Rosenfeld (1988), for example, emphasizes the battles between intensely personified, developmentally primitive good and bad objects. In particular, he finds conflicts between variously libidinized part objects derived from the paranoid-schizoid position and the masochistic patient's efforts to reconcile and integrate them into more advanced or whole representations characteristic of the depressive position. Bergler

(1961) added the importance that early pain can play in self-definition so that some masochistic children will seek it out in order to counteract their otherwise difficult-to-manage symbiotic longings. "Cutters," that is, adolescents (usually girls) who self-mutilate, sometimes do so in order to defend against their unconscious longings to fuse. One must wonder if the occurrence of this symptom during adolescence is so common because of the complex conflicts stimulated by the teen-aged girl's efforts to separate from her mother. And Asch (1976) notes how the oppositionality and negativism of some masochistic patients involves their struggles against unconscious urges to fuse. Adult masochistic patients often play out this typical rapprochement or anal stage conflict in the transference, frequently leading to insidious and tenacious negative therapeutic reactions. But Sarah, the three-year-old girl who sparked my interest in this subject behaved similarly. Her negativism and oppositionality toward me was striking and has been described elsewhere (Sugarman, 1991a). It also resurfaced in termination: the most noteworthy time being immediately after we had formalized her termination plans. Thus, masochism as a defense against and attempt to modulate symbiotic yearnings can be an important dynamic to analyze.

As Asch (1976) mentions, it is "a special characterological defense against the regressive pull to symbiotic fusion" (p. 385) and demonstrates how early character traits develop. Dynamically, it often involves an "ambivalent identification with a depressed, pre-oedipal object" (Olinik, 1964, p. 545). In Sarah's and Bobby's cases, however, the ambivalent identification was with an angry and sexually overcharged, not depressed, mother. Regardless, the identification is an intense one that can be problematic to analyze. Sarah never formed the overt and direct libidinal attachment to me that usually occurs when analyzing children of this age because she defensively split her transference—her mother remained the good, idealized and beloved object while I often was the bad, devalued one. It was also quite apparent that she felt positively toward me, but she remained reluctant to acknowledge these feelings directly despite many attempts to analyze her defenses against them. Bobby, in contrast, did not split his transference. But his mother eventually terminated the analysis prematurely when she felt threatened by the loss of his sexualized, symbiotic attachment to her. It is not always only the masochistic child who struggles with managing primitive yearnings.

Narcissistic Contributors

The narcissistic contributors to masochism have been discussed for some time (e.g., Bergler, 1949). This emphasis should not be surprising given the importance of the superego in formulations about the subject. But it is only more recently that the narcissistic function of masochism has been appreciated from a more encompassing perspective that considers it in terms of other defensive and developmental factors including the importance of the ego ideal discussed above (Asch, 1976; Cooper, 1984, 1988; Novick and Novick, 1991, 1996; Stolorow, 1975). This expansion is particularly important to the emphasis of this chapter—that is, children, even very young ones, can suffer from masochistic symptoms and character traits because of issues that may arise before the oedipal stage of development and/or may have little to do with the unique conflict of that stage.

Cooper (1988), for example, stresses how narcissism and masochism have an early and complex developmental relationship that precedes the oedipal stage or its conflicts. In keeping with my beliefs, he says: "I suggest that a full appreciation of the roles of narcissism and masochism in development and in pathology requires that we relinquish whatever remains of what Freud referred to as the 'shibboleth' of the centrality of the Oedipus complex in neurosogenesis" (p. 117). In contrast, Cooper aligns his thinking with Bergler and emphasizes how 'infantile megalomania or omnipotence" is a developmentally early means to regulate anxiety. Self-directed pain then becomes a way to deny the frustrations, disappointments, etc., over which the young child feels anxiety about having no control. "Faced with unavoidable frustration, the danger of aggression against parents, who are also needed and loved, and the pain of self-directed aggression, the infant nonetheless attempts to maintain essential feelings of omnipotence and self-esteem" (p. 122). Displeasure is turned to pleasure to maintain an illusion of omnipotent control of self and others that assuages the anxiety associated with helplessness.

Gabriella, a ten-year-old girl brought for a consultation about her trichotillomania that was not being helped by SSRI medication offers a good example of this interaction between pain, narcissism and anxiety regulation. Her developmental history was noteworthy for her difficulties with affect regulation from her earliest days. Gabriella was described as unable to be soothed despite her parents' best efforts and consultations with experts. Anxiety had been a ubiquitous part of her life from the beginning. Stranger anxiety became separation anxiety that turned into social anxiety when she turned school-aged, etc. Cognitive-behavioral psychotherapy had failed in her early elementary school years, leading to a psychiatric consultation and the prescribing of SSRI medication. This helped with her social anxiety, only to be superseded by the hair pulling when she was eight years old. She was virtually bald and needed to wear a wig by the time I saw her. In addition, she was so anxious about school work that special tutors were needed to sit with her and help her with projects and homework in the subjects that made her anxious, despite having been tested as having an IQ over 140. Gabriella was also afraid to sleep by herself or even to be upstairs in her house unless an adult was with her.

Her developmental history suggested longstanding internal conflicts over aggression leading to inhibited separation-individuation strivings. Her father was opposed to psychoanalysis but agreed to twice weekly psychotherapy with the understanding that we would reconsider if Gabriella did not show symptomatic improvement in a reasonable period of time. In addition, the parents understood that symptomatic improvement was not the only goal and that Gabriella's masochistic symptom placed her at risk of more serious problems during adolescence if her underlying conflicts and structural vulnerabilities were not attenuated.

Gabriella began her psychotherapy by agreeing with my suggestion that her hair pulling seemed to soothe her. Realizing this seemed to mobilize her interest in understanding her own mind and its workings. Thus, we focused on her inordinate difficulty with affect regulation and inability to use her mind to regulate it. She grasped that she used externalizing and self-injurious behavior to regulate her emotions in the only way she could. Slowly and carefully we examined the emotions that were the most difficult for her, the ways that she attempted unsuccessfully to regulate them, the causes for them, the anxiety that accompanied them and strategies to gain greater comfort. Anger was highlighted early on, and we worked to gain greater comfort with it. Putting it into words and becoming comfortable with fantasizing ways to express it toward those who angered her was a useful early strategy. As this occurred, she became able to be aware of and to express her anger with less conflict and anxiety. Her hair pulling gradually stopped, and her hair grew back so that she no longer needed a wig. This symptomatic success encouraged more curiosity into her mind's workings. The work that ensued has led recently into her awareness of her inordinate need to control others in an effort to control her emotions that seem so frightening and overpowering to her. Thus, she left a session recently telling her mother that our work had led her to realize: "I'm a control freak!" This work, still in progress, demonstrates the intimate connection of pain being used in the service of underlying affect and narcissistic regulation. As Gabriella became aware of her problems with affect regulation and use of self-directed aggression to counteract frustration and helplessness, she gave up her self-mutilating behavior. Its partial recurrence during a recent, serious illness of her father's highlights her continuing masochistic vulnerability as well as the more general relationship between narcissistic vulnerability and masochism in childhood.

The Novicks (Novick and Novick, 1991, 1996) have more recently brought the narcissistic determinants of masochism into focus with their emphasis on what they call the delusion of omnipotence. "In our studies of masochistic patients, we have found derivatives of each phase, but, like a thread linking knots of fixation points at oral, anal, and phallic-oedipal phases, there is a delusion of omnipotence that infuses the patients' past and current functioning" (1996, pp. 49–50). Like Cooper, they note the defensive aspect of masochistic omnipotence that involves aggressive fantasies of complete domination of others accompanied by an incessant refusal to accept reality limitations. But they also stress that the resulting omnipotence can lead to ego defects. Masochistic children and adults are similar in the degree to which they go to deny such constraints, a degree that can seriously disrupt reality testing. Lawrence, a twelve-year-old boy whom I was analyzing because of his intense control struggles and rage outbursts with his parents and teachers (Sugarman, 1994), showed this characteristic omnipotence. He regularly vented to me how "unfair" it was that his parents or teachers were allowed to make decisions about, and exercise control over, him. It was impossible during his early sessions to persuade him to step back and reflect on how unrealistic he was being in his demands that his opinions have an equal weight to those of his parents. There was no legitimate reason that children should not have equal rights with adults from his perspective. To him, this seemed a serious omission from the constitution of the United States. At these moments he seemed to lose his observing ego. Confrontation, humor, or questioning him about the admitted lack of such preoccupation shown by his friends were of little avail in assuaging his sense of narcissistic injury and sense of entitlement.

His omnipotence also appeared in the transference wherein he routinely denied the correctness of any of my interpretations or confrontations if they differed with his perceptions of how the world, others and most importantly, he, himself, worked. In desperation, I finally pointed out his frequent reports to me that his parents said that I was the best child psychoanalyst in San Diego, a view that he consciously supported. "I must have everyone, including you, fooled if I'm wrong as often as you say I am." Only the cognitive dissonance of having his narcissistically valued idealization of me challenged had any impact on his omnipotent oppositionality and belief that he was always correct in any disagreement.

In contrast, Phillip, an early adolescent seen during his high school years, showed similar grandiosity (Sugarman, 2011). His angry rants about his teachers and his parents ultimately gave way to analytic scrutiny of what we came to call his "chutzpah" factor. It was easier to foster self-reflection or insightfulness (Sugarman, 2003b, 2006) with him than with Lawrence. Nonetheless, it took some years of work, and countless unnecessary and self-destructive provocations of teachers, before he admitted and understood the dynamic reasons for this cherished belief in his superiority enough to bring it under control. Before this insightfulness occurred, Phillip strikingly resembled the Novicks' description of such pathology in adult analysands: "the image we get from analysts describing the omnipotent fantasies of adult patients is of a raging, hostile tyrant whose behavior is fueled by envy and is a compensation for feelings of helplessness and shame" (Novick and Novick, 1996, p. 51).

Like Gabriella, Phillip's developmental history revealed him to have been a difficult-to-soothe infant. It was impossible in his case to ascertain whether this reflected constitutional vulnerability or a compromised mother-infant match. His ADHD symptoms did suggest that he might have been born with a constitutional oversensitivity and hyperreactivity to internal and external stimuli. But his mother was also reported to be prone to rage attacks whenever frustrated. Regardless, both he and Gabriella ultimately suffered interference in the early pleasurable interaction between them and their mothers. "The infancy of the severely masochistic patients we have seen was marked by significant disturbances in the pleasure economy from birth" (Novick and Novick, 1996, p. 52). Such a disturbance ultimately leads the infant to feel ineffectual in eliciting needed or desired responses from their caretakers. Dysphoric and/or anxious affect results, along with an unconscious or occasionally conscious association between the representation of the caretaker and affective pain. Omnipotence and an imaginary world wherein they are all powerful become preferable to feeling incompetent and out of control. The Novicks note that toddlerhood is a particularly relevant developmental stage for masochism because of the toddler's normally exponential expansion of self-regulatory skills. To the degree that the toddler is unable to become competently self-regulating, a cycle of rage, guilt and blame ensues and the toddler is made to feel "omnipotently responsible for mother's pain, anger, helplessness, and inadequacy" (Novick and Novick, 1996, p. 54). This occurred with all the children discussed thus far except for Gabriella.

Aggressive Rather than Libidinal Issues

In contrast to the usual emphasis on oedipal libidinal conflicts in masochism, Rosenfeld (1988) and others (Novick and Novick, 1996) emphasize the role of intense early aggression and a failure to balance it with normal, libidinal feelings and pleasure. Healthy balancing of aggression with love and comfort usually occurs far earlier than the oedipal stage. In general, the histories of masochistic children reveal experiences in which the parents could not soothe or contain the child's normal or exaggerated aggression during their pre-oedipal years. Instead they tended to be critical, excessively controlling or helpless and blaming of their infants' or toddlers' aggression. Bobby's parents consistently complained he had always been more difficult and disruptive than his idealized older brother. Their blaming and subtly critical rejection led to aggression being turned against himself from early on. Prior to the apparently precipitating surgery, Bobby was reported to react to anger-provoking situations in play group by going to sleep instead of reacting aggressively. And his face was remarkably impassive during the evaluation while he displayed no age-appropriate excitement or exuberance, even after he had gotten to know me for several sessions. Inhibition of affect, particularly aggression, was striking, seemingly an indication of submission to a threatening and externalizing environment that the Novicks (Novick and Novick, 1996) find to characterize the toddlerhood of masochistic children. They believe such inhibition is a defensive attempt by the child to maintain an idealized representation of the mother and to keep her safe from the destructive rage of his or her anal sadism. Bobby's analytic material demonstrated this dynamic quite directly.

In general, my experience in analyzing children with masochistic psychopathology is that aggression, far more than sexuality, is the drive being managed and expressed through the masochistic symptom or character trait. This should not be surprising. Over twenty-five years ago, Chused (1988) noted how often aggression, not sexuality, characterizes the transference neuroses of children. The aggressive drive seems to play a far more prominent role in children's internal worlds, and subsequently their pathology, than is often appreciated. Interestingly, many analysts suggest that aggressive impulses play a greater role than libidinal ones in masochistic beating fantasies, also (e.g., Mahony, 1997; Shengold, 1997). At times, the child's defensive sexualization of his or her anger can disguise the underlying conflict, making it appear to be a sexual one (Sugarman, in press). But the analytic process with masochistic children usually reveals the sexuality to be defensive, and the child to have access to this particular defense because of parental overstimulation in the same way Coen (1992) finds to occur with adults. One must wonder if this defensive sexualization has been another contributor to the idea that true masochism requires oedipal conflicts. After all, it is this stage wherein infantile sexuality makes its most striking appearance. But once one realizes that the sexuality apparent in masochistic children is usually a defensive effort to cope with and regulate pre-oedipal aggression, it seems unnecessary to insist on tying masochism to the Oedipus complex.

The Importance of the Environment

The various masochistic children described above all experienced problems with parental attunement and soothing. Some had challenging temperaments that required a far better than expectably empathic parent to cope with it. Others had parents who showed minimal empathy or capacity to calm their child. Still others were born at times that their parents were unusually unavailable (e.g., suffering a post partum depression). Regardless of the reason for the lack of attunement, masochism in children does not seem to occur just out of normative developmental conflicts (Nagera, 1966) or from unconscious fantasies associated with what has been traditionally called an infantile neurosis. My clinical experience indicates that the environment always plays a significant role in the pathogenesis of masochism, in contrast to other childhood symptoms that may arise from internal conflicts with minimal input from it. This should not be surprising if one accepts the thesis that masochism in children and adolescents usually involves mental structures or functions that have gone awry. That is, masochistic symptoms and character traits always, in part, involve an attempt to regulate certain internal states that are particularly difficult to modulate or tolerate. An excessively critical superego, an ego ideal distorted by the quality of the introjects that comprise it, difficulties with affect and/or narcissistic regulation, or a preponderance of developmentally primitive aggression over libidinal strivings usually implicate the environment as playing a major etiological role. This is even more likely the case when the child is young. Parental failure to attune to and soothe the young infant leads to the kind of problems with self-regulation that characterize the masochistic children and adolescents described in this chapter. "At times the mother fails in this role, and the infant's tensions escalate. This may be because of a deficiency of the infant, or because mother herself is emotionally unavailable. . . . The infant may then experience persistent and diffuse tension states. Instead of fostering self-regulation, the persistent distress predisposes the infant to self-regulatory disorders" (Tyson, 1996b, p. 177). A similar need for sensitive and attuned parenting occurs throughout the child's and adolescent's development. It promotes the internalization of the many self-regulating functions that contribute to a developmentally mature level of mental organization capable of adapting to the world beyond the parents (Sugarman and Jaffe, 1990). But the masochistic children and adolescents described above did not receive such parenting. Usually beginning in infancy, and continuing up to the time of the consultation (and, at times, even after the treatment ended), their parents seemed unable find ways to help them learn to self-regulate.

The misattuned parenting received by Sarah (Sugarman, 2008) and Bobby (Sugarman, 2003a) has been described elsewhere. Thus, I will use Lawrence (Sugarman, 1994) as another example of the role that parents seem to have in the pathogenesis of masochism. He was born with a serious illness that necessitated his remaining in the hospital for the first two months of his life. This inauspicious beginning was further complicated by the career ambitions of his well meaning but high achieving parents. Thus, he received even less parental cuddling and comforting than many of the other newborns in his neonatal nursery. When he could come home, his mother simply could not adapt to the developmental difficulties caused by his illness and traumatic birth. These difficulties were not severe but they did make him a "not easy" baby. The parents' tone when describing these days to me was one of mildly sarcastic derision and a subtle blaming of Lawrence for having been so difficult. Things did not improve as he developed. Despite being quite bright, his peer relations were always problematic because of his temper and lack of consideration for the other children. Descriptions of his home life made it clear that regulation of anger was a problem for the entire family, not just for Lawrence. Household life sounded like a war zone with parents screaming at children, children screaming at each other and their parents, and a sense that no one regulated affects except through psychosomatic symptoms or masochistic provocation.

Narcissistic regulation was also difficult for Lawrence. His good grades were never good enough for his parents who were preoccupied from his conception with him attending their alma mater. Sports were quite difficult for him, a serious socialization problem for a boy in southern California; he was not athletically inclined and had always had difficulty with both gross and fine motor coordination. Furthermore, his intense and poorly contained rage caused such conflict that sports involving physical contact were so anxiety provoking that he could not perform well. Tennis became the sport he would play as his high school required all students to participate in a competitive sport or in physical education classes. The latter were so humiliating for Lawrence that he preferred to languish on the junior varsity team bench in perpetuity rather than attend the classes. And playing tennis with his father was one of the rare opportunities for them to potentially interact in ways that did not lead to power struggles. Unfortunately though, well into adolescence, his father could not use this opportunity to help Lawrence learn to regulate his anger, his narcissistic vulnerability, or just to have a positive interaction that might balance out the usual negative ones. Thus, the patient described their usual matches to me as situations wherein his father showed no concept of allowing Lawrence any sense of the pride or competence that comes with occasionally besting one's father in direct competition. Never did Lawrence win a set against his father in the entire duration of the analysis. If he played in the backcourt to return his father's powerful ground strokes, his father dropped short shots just over the net and laughed at Lawrence's futile charges forward in an attempt to return the ball. If he played close to the net to counteract this strategy, his father slammed the ball directly at him, more than occasionally hitting him or more often leading to the ball caroming off Lawrence's racket and out of bounds.

I struggled with my own countertransference indignation at the father's sadism and insensitivity as I tried to help Lawrence realize, acknowledge, and manage his hurt, disappointment, humiliation, and rage. Over the course of a seven year analysis he became adept at finding adaptive compromise formations as he gave up his masochistic ones. But the parents' behavior never improved during that time. This is not uncommon in my experience. Despite my belief in the importance of meeting with parents often, and working actively with them to improve their relationship with their child, the parents of the masochistic children I have treated are remarkably tenacious in their lack of attunement. Exceptions do occur. Sarah's mother was one. But the environment's contribution to this sort of pathology tends to be more prominent and resistant to change than what occurs in many other types of childhood problems.

CONCLUSION

In conclusion, it is my experience that the artificial and false dichotomy between masochism and protomasochism made when discussing childhood psychopathology confuses and obfuscates the essential nature and function of this disorder. This distinction is a remnant of the topographic emphasis on drive based conflicts leading to unconscious fantasies that cause psychopathological symptoms and character problems. Specifically it harkens back to Freud's belief that the Oedipus complex and its attendant conflicts are the direct cause of symptom and character neuroses (Sugarman, 2007). As such it perpetuates a "developmental lag" in integrating the tenets of his structural model into clinical understanding as it pertains both to diagnosis and to technique. Contemporary structural and/or ego psychological thinkers have spent the last decade and one-half trying to correct for this lag by reformulating diagnostic and technical concepts to account for the conceptual implications and advantages offered by the tripartite model of id, ego, and superego. Regardless of whether one finds the structural model or the ego psychological one more helpful in organizing clinical data, analysts using these theoretical models have gone far beyond postulating the drive developmental line and the conflicts that it gives rise to, most notably the oedipal conflict, as the major or sole contributor to pathogenesis. As ego and superego development gain equal stature and prominence in contributing to normal and pathological mental functioning, modern Freudian psychoanalysts are being forced to rethink many so-called shibboleths. The centrality of the Oedipus complex in explaining psychopathology and guiding psychoanalytic technique is one that is being increasingly questioned (Brown and Sugarman, 2002).

The problems that ensue when rigidly insisting that the pathogenesis of masochism involves oedipal conflicts have been noted for over one half of a century. Yet current day psychoanalytic curricula and readings continue to use Freud's mostly topographic papers on the subject to conceptualize it as just one more psychoneurosis, this time involving the linking of self-punishment to pleasure out of unconscious guilt over incestuous oedipal strivings. Even in his last paper on the subject, Freud (1924) used his recently articulated superego construct to explain the masochistic patient's guilt over such strivings. Pre-oedipal issues and conflicts received minimal consideration while the notion of masochistic phenomena being a means to compensate for structural difficulties merited even less. Despite the voluminous literature challenging this limited model that flies in the face of Waelder's (1936) concept of multiple function, it prevailed, in part, because the preponderance of this literature focused on analytic experience with adult patients. Because it is impossible to grow into adulthood without engaging the challenges and conflicts of the oedipal stage, masochistic adults, of course, demonstrate oedipal residue in their analytic material. Consequently it is not a far leap, and does not require straying far from the clinical data, to conclude that oedipal dynamics and conflicts are significant contributors to the masochistic phenomena receiving analytic scrutiny.

But the picture becomes more complicated once one examines the analytic data and developmental histories of children and adolescents being psychoanalyzed for masochistic symptoms and character traits. The Novicks (1996) are the most prominent of many child analysts who have noted the importance of pre-oedipal experiences and conflicts in the creation of such phenomena. The patients described in this chapter all demonstrate the unusually significant role of the parents in the development of masochistic psychopathology during childhood. Each of the children and adolescents described began life with a far less than optimal or average expectable parent-infant interaction. Tyson (1996b) eloquently describes the cascading impact of early failures in mother-infant attunement regardless of the constitutional versus environmental balance in causing it.

> The diffuse tension states of early infancy evolve into diffuse anxiety and/or primitive rage states that may interfere with the infant's being able to experience the mother's libidinal investment. This quickly leads to a distortion of the maternal introject, and ordinary developmental, phase-specific conflicts become intensified and distorted. . . . The conflicts of the anal-rapprochement phase, for example, easily become exaggerated and intensified. Aggression leads to marked ambivalence and object relations become distorted and organized around sado-masochistic fantasies. (p. 184)

Such difficulties only spiral throughout the child's subsequent development as parents and child find each other's company distressing and frustrating. As a result, important self-regulatory functions usually internalized out of a comfortable and safe parent-child attachment fail to become solidly entrenched as stable mental functions and structures. To be sure, internal conflict plays a significant role in masochistic symptoms and character traits as soon as there is enough cognitive development for defenses and fantasies to occur. But the intensity of these conflicts, particularly the sadistic rage that characterizes them, derives from early failures by the parents to find ways to promote experiences of safety and comfort in the interaction with their child.

The Novicks (Novick and Novick, 2003, 2004) have this point in mind in their idea of two systems of self-regulation. Their experience with masochistic patients who cling to their masochistic ways of experiencing the world, and resist the analyst's attempts to help them to change, led them to realize how important such patients' masochism is in regulating self-esteem. Thus, the masochistic individual actualizes, in the transference, his or her "closed, omnipotent, sadomasochistic system, in which the active search for pain and suffering has transformed experiences of helplessness into a hostile defense" (Novick and Novick, 1999, p. 1). Both they (Novick and Novick, 2004) as well as Tyson (1996b) emphasize that the rigid and punitive superego found in masochistic patients involves a defensive grandiosity far more than it involves guilt over oedipal longings. One former analysand would routinely castigate herself for multiple childhood transgressions that she believed caused her parents to have been, as well to presently be, so cruel, critical and rejecting toward her. Any of my attempts to engage her curiosity about her vitriolic condemnation of herself for relatively benign "sins" (such as asking her stay-at-home mom to drive her to ballet class during early adolescence) led to rageful attacks of me for my "nice guy" approach to psychoanalysis. She believed she needed an analyst like that of a friend on the east coast who would "hold my feet to the fire!" Finally, I was able to interpret the grandiosity underlying these superego attacks as a defense against facing the narcissistic limitations of her parents and accepting that she would never receive the sort of parenting for which she longed. Insisting that her own "bad" behavior was the cause of their attitudes toward her maintained the fantasy that they would become loving if she only modified her behavior. Sadistic self-torment felt preferable to the helplessness that accompanied accepting that she could never change or control her parents.

From this perspective the structure of the superego has become compromised so that its functioning in terms of facilitating self-regulation is undermined. Sarah, Bobby, and Lawrence all had superegos so punitive and unyielding that it first had to be modified via analysis before insightfulness in the service of self-regulation could occur. As with the above described patient, self-reflection could not occur until the patient's "masochistic delusion of omnipotence" (Novick and Novick, 1991, 1996) had been addressed.

> For the child to develop the ego split . . . and self-observation essential for working analytically, he or she must have sufficiently neutralized the aggressive-sadistic nature of his or her superego to examine mental processes without experiencing narcissistic depletion. Otherwise, self-other differentiation and self-reflection become compromised by conflict. (Sugarman, 1994, p. 332)

Parents of masochistic children and adolescents do not allow themselves to be used by the developing child as comforters or organizers. Rather than functioning as auxiliary egos and fostering a sense of safety, they fan the flames of the child's anxiety and interfere with it serving a signal function to stimulate effective defense and self-responsibility. "When young children are not able to 'use' their parents in the manner Winnicott described, superego development is delayed and impaired. Such children frequently become preoccupied with narcissistic issues related to omnipotent demands for control and/or domination" (Tyson, 1996b, p. 186). Externalization and blaming of others while feeling unfairly victimized alternates with vicious attacks on themselves and a variety of masochistic behaviors and provocations. Rather than a mature superego capable of generating just enough guilt to signal the need to control themselves before transgressing, masochistic children develop a superego that is both ineffectual and tyrannical (Novick and Novick, 2004). Sadistic attacks on themselves become common, but usually after the fact. It is as though the purpose of the superego is to make the child feel terrible rather than to help him or her to regulate him or herself so that he or she does not have to feel guilty, let alone reprehensible. But this pain unconsciously feels preferable to having to deal with the masochistic child's overwhelming hurt, disappointment, and anxiety at having to face his or her own powerlessness to make the environment different.

If the treatment of such children goes well, they eventually come to accept the irony that effective self-regulation can only happen once they accept their helplessness to change their parents or important others. Sarah, the three-year-old girl who was the original impetus for this chapter, poignantly demonstrated this irony and how difficult it is to accept at the onset of the termination phase of her analysis (Sugarman, 1991b). Immediately after finalizing the details of her termination process following several session of work, she expressed anxiety about the pierced earring holes in her ears becoming infected. I reminded her about previous insights into her somatizing and wondered if it reflected feeling worried about not seeing me anymore once she terminated. "I don't care about seeing you, I don't even like you," Sarah replied. "Not liking me will certainly help you not miss me," I said. At that point, Sarah angrily retorted, "I can stop whenever I want and I can walk out and stop now!" We managed to work our way through this reemergence of her omnipotent defense that had brought her into analysis. But its immediate reemergence around the prospect of ultimately losing me highlights how difficult it is for masochistic children to accept and tolerate their helplessness without resorting to this self-destructive defense.

It also demonstrates the degree to which masochistic symptoms and character traits in children and adolescents are primarily attempts to self regulate. The failure of their early and formative parental interactions to promote effective ways to manage their feelings, self-esteem, and impulses leads them to fall back on pathological and self-destructive ways of doing so. Hence, such symptoms and character traits in childhood involve more than traditional compromise formations. They also involve faulty mental structures and functions. Unconscious fantasies do develop to explain such impairments. But these fantasies should not be viewed as the primary contributor to pathogenesis. Unlike many other childhood problems, unconscious fantasies and the compromise formations that contribute to them are not the primary causal factor. Instead masochistic symptoms and character traits arise from early and ongoing problems with parental attunement that disrupts the healthy internalization process that promotes mature and adaptive self-regulation. Thus, masochistic psychopathology in children and adolescents involves far more than neurotic conflicts over oedipal longing. They help such children to regulate emotions, self-esteem, and ultimately themselves to compensate for early and less than optimal failures to internalize and develop more adaptive ways to do so.

REFERENCES

Asch, S. S. (1976). Varieties of negative therapeutic reaction and problems of technique. *Journal of the American Psychoanalytic Association* 24: 383–408.

——— (1980). Beating fantasy: Symbiosis and child battering. *International Journal of Psychoanalytic Psychotherapy* 8: 653–58.

——— (1988). The analytic concepts of masochism: A reevaluation. In *Masochism: Current Psychoanalytic Perspectives*, eds. R. A. Glick and D. I. Meyers. Hillsdale, NJ: Analytic Press, 93–116.

Bergler, E. (1948). Further studies on beating fantasies. *Psychoanalytic Quarterly* 22: 480–86.

——— (1949). *The Basic Neurosis, Oral Regression and Psychic Masochism*. New York: Grune & Stratton.

——— (1961). *Curable and Incurable Neurosis—Problems of Neurotic vs. Malignant Masochism*. New York: Liveright.

Berliner, B. (1947). On some psychodynamics of masochism. *Psychoanalytic Quarterly* 16: 322–33.

Brown, J., and Sugarman, A. (2002). The Oedipus complex. In *The Encyclopedia of Psychotherapy*, eds. M. Hersen and W. Sledge. New York: Academic Press, 715–19.

Burgner, M., and Kennedy, H. (1980). Different types of sado-masochistic behavior in children. *Dialogue* 4: 50–59.

Busch, F. (1995). *The Ego at the Center of Clinical Technique*. Northvale, NJ: Jason Aronson.

Chused, J. F. (1988). The transference neurosis in child analysis. *Psychoanalytic Study of the Child* 43: 51–81.

Colarusso, C. A. (1992). *Child and Adult Development: A Psychoanalytic Introduction for Clinicians*. New York: Plenum.

Coen, S. J. (1992). *The Misuse of Persons: Analyzing Pathological Dependency*. Hillsdale, NJ: Analytic Press.

Cooper, A. M. (1984). The unusually painful analysis: A group of narcissistic-masochistic characters. In *Psychoanalysis: The Vital Issues*, eds. G. H. Pollock and J. E. Gedo. New York: International Universities Press, 45–67.

——— (1988). The narcissistic-masochistic character. In *Masochism: Current Psychoanalytic Perspectives*, eds. R. A. Glick and D. I. Meyers. Hillsdale, NJ: Analytic Press, 117–38.

Fenichel, O. (1945). *The Psychoanalytic Theory of Neurosis*. New York: Norton.

Ferber, L., and Gray, P. (1966). Beating fantasies, clinical and theoretical considerations. *Bulletin of the Philadelphia Psychoanalytic Association of Psychoanalysis* 16: 186–206.

Freud, S. (1919). A child is being beaten. *Standard Edition* 17: 175–204.

—— (1923). The ego and the id. *Standard Edition* 19: 12–66.

—— (1924). The economic problem of masochism. *Standard Edition* 19: 157–70.

Galenson, E. (1980). Preoedipal determinants of a beating fantasy. *International Journal of Psychoanalytic Psychotherapy* 8: 649–52.

—— (1988) The precursors of masochism: Protomasochism. In *Masochism: Current Psychoanalytic Perspectives*, eds. R. A. Glick and D. I. Meyers. Hillsdale, NJ: Analytic Press, 189–204.

Glenn, J. (1984a). A note on loss, pain, and masochism in children. *Journal of the American Psychoanalytic Association* 32: 63–73.

—— (1984b). Psychic trauma and masochism. *Journal of the American Psychoanalytic Association* 32: 357–86.

—— (1989). From protomasochism to masochism: A developmental view. *Psychoanalytic Study of the Child* 44: 73–86.

Glick, R. A., and Meyers, D. I. (1988). Introduction. In *Masochism: Current Perspectives*, eds. R. A. Glick and D. I. Meyers. Hillsdale, NJ: Analytic Press, 1–25.

Gray, P. (1994). *The Ego and the Analysis of Defense*. Northvale, NJ: Jason Aronson.

Grossman, W. I. (1986). Notes on masochism: A discussion of the history and development of a psychoanalytic concept. *Psychoanalytic Quarterly* 55: 379–413.

Holder, A. (1982). Preoedipal contributors to the formation of the superego. *Psychoanalytic Study of the Child* 37: 245–72.

Kernberg, O. (1988). Clinical dimensions of masochism. In *Masochism: Current Psychoanalytic Perspectives*, eds. R. A. Glick and D. I. Meyers. Hillsdale, NJ: Analytic Press, 61–80.

Lester, M. (1957). An unconscious beating fantasy. *International Journal of Psychoanalysis* 38: 22–31.

Mahony, P. J. (1997). "A Child Is Being Beaten": A clinical, historical, and textual study. In *On Freud's "A Child Is Being Beaten,"* eds. E. S. Person. New Haven: Yale University Press, 47–66.

Maleson, F. G. (1984). The multiple meanings of masochism in psychoanalytic discourse. *Journal of the American Psychoanalytic Association* 32: 325–56.

Modell, A. H. (1997). Humiliating fantasies and the pursuit of unpleasure. In *On Freud's "A Child Is Being Beaten,"* ed. E. S. Person. New Haven: Yale University Press, 67–75.

Myers, W. (1980). The psychodynamics of a beating fantasy. *International Journal of Psychoanalytic Psychotherapy* 8: 623–38.

Nagera, H. (1966). *Early Childhood Disturbances, the Infantile Neurosis, and the Adulthood Disturbances*. New York: International Universities Press.

Novick, J., and Novick, K. K. (1972). Beating fantasies in children. *International Journal of Psychoanalysis* 53: 237–42.

—— (1991). Some comments on masochism and the delusion of omnipotence from a developmental perspective. *Journal of the American Psychoanalytic Association* 39: 307–28.

—— (1996). *Fearful Symmetry: The Development and Treatment of Sadomasochism*. Northvale, NJ: Jason Aronson.

—— (1999). *Two Systems of Self-Regulation Regulation*. Paper presented at the 88th Annual Meeting of the American Psychoanalytic Association. May 1999.

—— (2004). The superego and the two-system model. *Psychoanalytic Inquiry* 24: 232–56.

Novick, K. K., and Novick, J. (1987). The essence of masochism. *Psychoanalytic Study of the Child* 42: 353–84.

—— (2003). Two systems of self-regulation and the differential application of psychoanalytic technique. *American Journal of Psychoanalysis* 63: 1–20.

Olinik, S. L. (1964). The negative therapeutic reaction. *International Journal of Psychoanalysis* 45: 540–48.

Rosenfeld, H. A. (1988). On masochism: A theoretical and clinical approach. In *Masochism: Current Psychoanalytic Perspectives*, eds. R. A. Glick and D. I. Meyers. Hillsdale, NJ: Analytic Press, 151–74.

Rubenfine, D. (1965). On beating fantasies. *International Journal of Psychoanalysis* 46: 315–22.

Sarnoff, C. A. (1988). Adolescent masochism. In *Masochism: Current Psychoanalytic Perspectives*, eds. R. A. Glick and D. I. Meyers. Hillsdale, NJ: Analytic Press, 205–24.

Schmideberg, M. (1948). On fantasies of being beaten. *Psychoanalytic Review* 35: 303–8.

Shengold, L. (1997). Comments of Freud's "A Child Is Being Beaten": A contribution to the study of the origin of sexual perversions. In *On Freud's "A Child Is Being Beaten,"* ed. E. S. Person. New Haven: Yale University Press, 76–94.

Stolorow, R. D. (1975). The narcissistic function of masochism and sadism. *International Journal of Psychoanalysis* 56: 441–48.

Sugarman, A. (1991a). Developmental antecedents of masochism: Vignettes from the analysis of a 3-year-old girl. *International Journal of Psychoanalysis* 72: 107–16.

——— (1991b). Termination of psychoanalysis with an early latency girl. In *Saying Goodbye: Termination in Child Psychoanalysis*, ed. A. Schmukler. Hillsdale, NJ: Analytic Press, 5–25.

——— (1994). Helping child analysands observe mental functioning. *Psychoanalytic Psychology* 11: 329–39.

——— (1999). The boy in the iron mask: Superego issues in the analysis of a 2-year-old encopretic. *Psychoanalytic Quarterly* 58: 497–519.

——— (2003a). Dimensions of the child analyst's role as a developmental object: Affect regulation and limit setting. *Psychoanalytic Study of the Child* 58: 189-213.

——— (2003b). A new model for conceptualizing insightfulness in the analysis of young children. *Psychoanalytic Quarterly* 72: 325–55.

——— (2006). Mentalization, insightfulness, and therapeutic action: the importance of mental organization. *International Journal of Psychoanalysis* 87: 965–87.

——— (2007). Whatever happened to neurosis? Who are we analyzing? And how?: The importance of mental organization. *Psychoanalytic Psychology* 24: 409–28.

——— (2008). The use of play to promote insightfulness in the analysis of children suffering from cumulative trauma. *Psychoanalytic Quarterly* 77: 799–833.

——— (2011). Thinking about attention deficit/hyperactivity disorder. *Richard e Piggle. Studi Psicoloanalitici del Bambino e dell' adolescente* 19: 134–50

——— (In press). The centrality of beating fantasies in the analysis of a three-year-old girl. *Psychoanalytic Inquiry*.

Sugarman, A., and Jaffe, L. S. (1990). Toward a developmental understanding of the self schema. *Psychoanalysis and Contemporary Thought* 13: 117–38.

Tyson, P. (1996a). Neurosis in childhood and in psychoanalysis: A developmental reformulation. *Journal of the American Psychoanalytic Association* 44: 143–65.

——— (1996b). Object relations, affect management, and psychic structure formation: The concept of object constancy. *Psychoanalytic Study of the Child* 51: 172–89.

Tyson, P., and Tyson, R. L. (1984). Narcissism and superego development. *Journal of the American Psychoanalytic Association* 32: 75–98.

——— (1990). *Psychoanalytic Theories of Development: An Integration*. New Haven: Yale University Press.

Tyson, R. L. (1983). Some narcissistic consequences of object loss. *Psychoanalytic Quarterly* 52: 205–24.

Valenstein, A. F. (1973). On attachment to painful feelings and the negative therapeutic reaction. *Psychoanalytic Study of the Child* 28: 365–92.

Waelder, R. (1936). The principle of multiple function: Observations on overdetermination. *Psychoanalytic Quarterly* 5: 45–62.

THREE

Some Suggestions for Engaging with the Clinical Problem of Masochism

Kerry Kelly Novick and Jack Novick, PhD

Nineteen-year-old Nick came for an evaluation because he found university an extremely painful experience even though he had little difficulty handling the academic demands. He was the second of three children in a middle-class family. He had few friends, no girlfriends and seemed tortured by guilt and despair. He felt that he had wasted his whole adolescence on drugs and alcohol, had not learned any social skills and had no idea what he wanted to do with the rest of his life. He felt lost, confused and in pain. Nick ended up in late adolescence with an omnipotent belief in suicide as his solution to his difficulties.

As he began analysis, he was unable to tolerate lying on the couch for fear of attack. When he moved to the chair, he was intensely uncomfortable with our mutual gaze and would grimace as if he were in physical pain. I was puzzled and confused[1] and also found it uncomfortable to be with him. This experience highlights a difficulty of work with people like Nick, whose lives are organized around pain and suffering (Novick, K. K. and Novick, J., 1987).

As our views have evolved, we have found that sadism and masochism are always connected; the bridge is the formation of magical omnipotent beliefs as a major defense against helplessness. In the course of development a "vicious cycle" (Wurmser, 1996, 2007) is created where masochistic suffering entitles the person to be an exception to the rules of society, reality, and biology and justifies acting on a sadistic omnipotent belief in the power to control the lives of others (Freud, 1916). But such behavior has to be continually justified by seeking out masochistic suffer-

51

ing and then finding victims for renewed sadistic attack. Thus we do not speak of sadism or masochism, but rather use the term sadomasochism to encompass the combined phenomena.

Sadomasochistic patients have long and arduous treatments. One characteristic of sadomasochism is that there is much drama, much apparent activity, but the goal is to avoid any change. One patient described it as his "big hamster exercise wheel. There is a lot of noise and activity but it just goes nowhere." This pathology is tenacious and strengths are often hard to initially discern, nurture, and sustain.

In our experience all patients present with troubled power dynamics in their personality functioning. From our clinical work on the tenacity of sadomasochistic power relationships and the defensive omnipotent beliefs and fantasies that organize them we have postulated two systems of self-regulation and conflict resolution. One system, the open system, is attuned to reality and characterized by joy, competence, and creativity. The other, the closed system, avoids reality and is characterized by power dynamics, omnipotence, and stasis.

In closed-system functioning, relationships have a sadomasochistic pattern; the psyche is organized according to magical, omnipotent beliefs; hostile, painful feelings and aggressive, self-destructive behavior cycle repeatedly with no real change or growth. Omnipotent beliefs are invoked as the main defensive self-protection. Externalization, denial and avoidance are used to support those beliefs. The aim is to control the other rather than change the self. Reality-based pleasure is experienced as a threat to omnipotent beliefs, since the closed system depends on feeling victimized. Pain is central to the closed system, as a means for attachment, defense, and gratification. Ego functions are co-opted in the service of maintaining omnipotent defenses and beliefs. Executive functions of the ego are stunted or resisted to preserve the conviction that achievements are quick, easy and result from forcing, rather than work. Rules of any sort, from the laws of physics to the conventions of society and the patterns of games, are undermined and denied. Children operating in the closed system feel like entitled exceptions to the parameters of reality.

A major contribution of psychoanalysis was to recognize the ego's experience of helplessness as traumatic. Anna Freud underscored that a major anxiety in adolescence is the fear of being overwhelmed by the instincts, a fear of the quantity rather than quality of instincts. In the Discussions on her "Ego and the Mechanisms of Defense" (Sandler and A. Freud, 1983), she elaborated on the idea that fear of helplessness underlies all the other anxieties in the classical sequence. We, along with Freud and all other subsequent developmental psychologists, see mastery as a fundamental human need. The opposite of mastery is helplessness in relation to inner and outer forces. But we differentiate between closed, omnipotent, sadomasochistic modes of mastery and open, competent methods.

The aim of self-regulation is the same in both systems. In the open system the maximum use of one's genuine mental and physical capacities to be realistically effective and competent is the method of mastering inner and outer forces. In the closed system the basis for mastery is omnipotent belief in the power and necessity to be a perpetrator or victim in order to survive. Developmental researchers speak of "multifinality" and "equifinality" to underscore the many varied pathways and diverse outcomes of developmental pathology (Cicchetti and Rogosch, 1996). We have emphasized the unifying theme of consolidation of closed-system omnipotent solutions at adolescence. Therefore conflicts in adolescence offer a window into all sadomasochistic functioning, whether we are studying children or adults. This also confirms the importance of addressing adolescent issues in the treatment of adults.

Closed-system functioning, with its omnipotent core beliefs, is the major obstacle in the transition from late adolescence to adulthood. Each of the sadomasochistic strands from earlier levels can be intensified under the impact of the real changes of adolescence. All of the developmental tasks of adolescence require a transformation of the relation to reality and fantasy, as part of the integration of the mature body and self. In the course of this integration, the normal adolescent achieves a new harmony of the pleasure and reality principles. For the adolescent operating in the closed system, the two remain in opposition, so that what is real is not pleasurable, and pleasure resides in unreal magical fantasies.

The resolution of the confrontation between the reality demands of adolescence and a person's omnipotent beliefs determines the outcome of adolescent development and sets the course for adult health or pathology. Clinging to the closed-system solution can lead to omnipotent self-sufficiency and avoidance of the adolescent process or an escalating series of self-destructive and hostile actions designed to deny reality, attribute responsibility and guilt to others, make others feel helpless and anxious, indeed to enact a magical sadomasochistic scenario of control over the feelings and actions of others. The transition to adulthood will then be blocked.

We will use the work with Nick as it unfolded through his treatment to illustrate our ideas about what was impeding his progression to adulthood and the techniques that supported his eventual development. We will look at the development of omnipotence and how hostile, magical beliefs figured in his repeated choice of closed-system solutions in the treatment and in his life. We suggest the techniques that helped Nick may be usefully applied in treatment at all ages.

CLOSED-SYSTEM DEVELOPMENTAL
UNDERPINNINGS AND DERIVATIVES

Infancy

We have suggested that pain-seeking behavior and attachment to pain are derived first from disturbances in the pleasure-pain economy in early mother-child interactions (Novick, K. K. and Novick, J., 1987; Novick, J. and Novick, K. K., 2007 [1996]). Derivatives from this level can appear in the form of an externalizing transference, where the analyst may experience pain, helplessness, or lack of attention or focus. Awareness that this may represent a re-creation of an early disturbance can help the analyst first bear and contain his responses to being rendered ineffective, stay open to the patient and eventually reconstruct the early addiction to pain. Through this work, the therapist will not only interpret the aggressive components in the interaction but can begin to identify the use of pain to maintain a tie to the other person.

Initially Nick's infancy and preschool years sounded unremarkable. There were apparently no potentially traumatic events such as major medical interventions or losses and so forth. However, as he settled into four-times-per-week treatment, he frequently became silent, squirmed and twisted on the couch and beat it with his fist, all with no apparent reason and no discernible precipitant. This confusing behavior went on for a while. Finally, I suggested that he might have experienced a very painful, confusing, and frustrating experience with his mother during infancy. I wondered if I were currently being made to feel what he had felt as an infant. Soon after, he told his mother what I had said. His mother could not respond directly, but walked out of the room and later wrote a letter to him. She told him that when he was a baby, she had felt unable to hold him, hug him, or tell him that she loved him. She had cared for his physical needs but then left him in his crib to cry himself to sleep. Nick's mother was the eldest child with a brother three years younger. In the mother's memory, the brother was adored, much loved and preferred. In the course of Nick's treatment we could explore together the probability that Nick represented the hated male rival who left her feeling abandoned and depressed.

Despite subsequent transformations, pain-seeking behavior represents an adaptation to what Stern has called "the actual shape of interpersonal reality" (1985, p. 255), or, as a patient said, "It's the smell of home." The role of parents and parent work is central to our understanding and technique of work with adolescents, even late adolescents (Novick, K. K. and Novick, J., 2005, 2013; Novick, J. and Novick, K. K., 2013). As DeVito (2009) suggests on the basis of attachment research, one can no longer exclude parents from treatment considerations in adolescent work. Their future impact on the child can be seen in how they react to the challenge of parenthood.

Nick's attachment to pain and his belief that pain alone connected him to needed people had its roots in his infancy. To us this early and persistent link between attachment and pain leads to an addiction to pain and what current neurological research calls a "brain trap" where usually separate brain centers get inextricably linked. A similar idea is "functional dystonia," where two distinct neurological loci get bonded by frequent repetition, like the index and middle fingers of classical guitarists (Doidge, 2007). As another late adolescent said, "Love walks with pain." But it takes more than a painful parent-child relationship in infancy or a disorganized attachment to maintain and consolidate the "brain trap" of pain and attachment, or the addiction to pain. The centrality of pain relative to pleasure continues through all the later phases of development.

Toddlerhood

Parents and children in toddlerhood are faced with the challenges of fusing aggression and love. When parents cannot contain and absorb aggression while retaining loving feelings, aggression can intensify and escalate for the child. The clinical ramifications of such an affective history are many: there may be a tendency in the treatment for both patient and therapist to be swamped by intense feelings that overwhelm the calm holding of the therapeutic setting. The analyst must find ways to maintain positive investment in the treatment and the patient and protect the good feelings and mutual respect of the relationship. This is especially important in work with angry and anguished late adolescent patients, who seem so effective in destroying the positive feelings in all their relationships. Adolescents who hurt themselves—whether by cutting, drug abuse, school failure or by abusive relationships—reproduce these efforts in treatment, destroying pleasure in understanding and mastery and denying the importance of the therapy and the therapist, often by missing sessions or coming late.

Nick was a very bright, active, curious and explorative toddler. He talked and walked by fourteen months and his parents described him as "into everything." Even in his late adolescence both parents did not see or minimized his older brother's persistent intense jealousy. Nick described him as "insanely jealous" and everything Nick did, even currently, was reacted to as a major attack on his older brother. The uncontrolled aggression of the older brother first emerged in the therapeutic relationship where Nick could not stay on the couch for fear I would attack him, then couldn't look at me while sitting in the chair for fear that I would see his critical or competitive thoughts and I would retaliate.

His parents seemed not to have any idea that the older brother's constant competitiveness had any effect on Nick. They first dismissed this as normal "sibling rivalry;" it took a full year of parent work to help the parents get in touch with their own sibling rivalries as children and, through those memories, begin to empathize with Nick's experience. As we worked on their transferences to Nick, it became clear that their negative feelings toward him as a second child may have begun even during his mother's pregnancy with him. They both then recalled how Nick began to do things secretively, not letting his brother see what he had done. Father recalled wondering why Nick was always so bland, as if he had to hide his feelings.

In Nick's sessions we began to see and reconstruct the sequence of feeling terrified of his brother and needing to hide his achievements and feelings. But then he began to feel special because he had the power to upset his brother. He transformed his pleasure in competent, creative functioning into an omnipotent belief in the power of his feelings and actions to "drive his brother crazy." Toddlers believe that physical power is commensurate with the intensity of their feelings. Nick's brother and parents confirmed this omnipotent belief.

This toddler experience can work its way into the transference relationship when the patient experiences every detail of the interaction with extreme intensity and may try to involve the analyst in the heightened excitement. Sometimes the patient insists vehemently that the analyst *must* agree with whatever he thinks—the intense feelings make it true. Despite the palpable presence of libidinal and aggressive elements, interpretation of the drive impulses is likely to leave the patient feeling attacked, criticized and vulnerable, and therefore prone to redouble hostile defenses and resistances. More ominously, interpretation at this point may take away the patient's only available defense and drive him to more regressed and malignant methods of control, such as paranoia or suicide (Blum, 1980). Before these drive impulses can safely be taken up, the analyst should first address the omnipotent belief in the overwhelming power of affects in its pervasive cognitive and emotional aspects.

A recurring omnipotent belief that persisted nearly to the end of his treatment was Nick's conviction that, if something bad happened, he was responsible and would be blamed. Early on, I had to cancel a session suddenly because of a family matter. When I returned the next week, Nick was convinced that I had left because he was "too much to handle." In the session before the one I had cancelled Nick had asked whether he were getting anywhere in his analysis. He was then certain that I had taken this as a criticism and had therefore refused to see him.

Here are two later examples of the persistence of Nick's toddler belief in the destructive power of his creativity and the need to hide successful actions from others while getting secret gratification. In his first position after graduating he was working on a new computer program which everyone needed but had difficulty using. For two weeks he stayed late at his job, worked out all the bugs in the program and circulated an un-signed document with instructions. Everyone was thrilled. The manager wanted to know who had done this outstanding work, but to this day no one knows. A bit later in his career he and three colleagues invented an award-winning technological advance and were being given the prize at a national convention. The four of them were on stage to receive the award, but only three could be seen. Nick was hiding behind the curtain.

In infancy pain became the signal and mode of attachment. In toddler-hood the joy of competent and creative achievements was corrupted and turned into a source of anxiety, frustration and helpless rage. Finally his brilliant mind became a hostile weapon to attack and humiliate his older brother and others. One of his earliest memories, dating back to before nursery school, was putting salt in the sugar bowl and watching his brother gag over what he thought would be a sweet cup of hot chocolate. He was sent home from preschool for having put glue on the children's chairs and coloring the water set out for a snack. Eventually he was expelled from two preschools before he was four because he was playing tricks on the other children and frightening them with monster tales he made up.

Phallic and Oedipal

Toward the end of the toddler period and entry to the phallic phase there is an important distinction to be mastered between assertion and aggression. Even in the best of circumstances, many parents confuse the two; the child's independence, exploration and curiosity may feel like too much for parents and they can respond as if the child is doing something assaultive. This then defines assertion as hostile and skews the child's own judgment about his autonomous actions.

In the period between four and six, Nick consolidated a harsh, tyran-nical conscience and his behavior oscillated between clever, sadistic at-tacks on others and sullen withdrawal and inhibition of function. He remembered thinking that he was a monster and then trying to justify his sadistic behavior. He thought about a neighbor girl who wanted to play with him. He would start playing and, as soon as the game became en-grossing, he would run away and leave the girl confused and frustrated. He recalled trying to find an excuse for this behavior, which gave him pleasure, but this was one of the few times he couldn't. After a while, the girl's mother refused to let the two children play together.

Nick's mother was clinically depressed and spent much time in a darkened room. Both parents blamed Nick, saying that he was too much for her and she needed to rest. Father was a brilliant and highly success-ful professional, but he was also intensely competitive and couldn't toler-ate being outdone by anyone. Nick recalled taking great delight in looking up facts and then asking his father questions, telling him when he was wrong. Father found it difficult to enjoy his son's brilliance and needed to be the best and the first at everything. This behavior remained unchanged into Nick's young adulthood and was a focus of much work with Nick and eventually with his father.

The infantile omnipotent belief in the power of pain to attach to others, the toddler belief in the omnipotence of angry thoughts and feelings, and the belief that normal assertion was omnipotently destructive were all internalized in the phallic-oedipal period in the form of a tyrannical superego out to destroy the self for pleasures (Novick, J. and Novick, K. K., 2005b). The pleasures included the ordinary sexual pleasures of the oedipal child, usually contained by the reality of loving parents. Additionally, in Nick's case his very existence was considered "too much," causing his mother to retreat into a darkened room. The delusion of omnipotence that is so central to closed-system functioning cannot be maintained without reality validation from the outside.

When he entered treatment at nineteen, Nick had never been in a love relationship of any kind with a woman or a man. It took years of work on his belief that his sexual desires were weird and destructive to enable him to begin talking to women. His first encounters were in fact rather sadistic as he would get a woman interested in him and then suddenly leave with no explanation. Nick's omnipotent conviction that his pleasures, including his sexuality, had caused his mother's depressive withdrawal and illness, led to his extreme inhibition. He tried to put his adolescent development on hold, rather than test his closed-system solutions against the reality of his own and others' feelings and reactions.

School-age

Ordinary reality correctives to closed-system constructs of the early phases were not effective as Nick moved into his school years. In fact, reality further confirmed his omnipotent destructiveness. Nick had few friends and he antagonized even those by disrupting cooperative play and making up games that only he could win. When he was about eight, his chronically depressed mother was hospitalized with a major depression and once again he was blamed for her condition.

Probably all three children were blamed, but Nick took the full responsibility and felt that his demandingness, selfishness, and sadism caused her to break down and need lengthy hospitalization. From then on, she was heavily medicated and had numerous rehospitalizations, all of which validated Nick's belief that he was an omnipotent, sadistic, destructive monster. The important latency tasks of developing pleasure in new skills and achievements, acknowledging the separateness of others by acceding to rules in play and interactions, and internalizing controls and sources of pleasure had not been accomplished.

Adolescence

The real adolescent changes in body, mind and social expectations are a challenge to all teenagers and many find an omnipotent solution to feelings of helplessness. Most, especially if supported by family and good friends, can draw on earlier open-system solutions, especially the latency establishment of competence and pleasure in reality. Nick had little of that to draw on. His parents were "soul blind" (Wurmser, 1994; Novick, J. and Novick, K. K., 2005a); they externalized and assigned blame for events which were either beyond anyone's capacity, like the mother's depression, or beyond Nick's capacity, like his brother's continued hostility which the parents should have dealt with years before. He had few friends and no girl friends, as he was terrified of hurting them. In mid-adolescence he maintained his hostile omnipotent defense by withdrawing completely into alcohol and marijuana. He found a few friends who shared an angry repudiation of all usual high school activities and, as he said, "my whole adolescence was spent in an alcoholic and drugged-up haze." His parents didn't seem to notice and the school tolerated his sporadic attendance since he was bright enough to get top grades with minimal work. He and his few friends were in a rage at everyone and felt justified in rejecting all expectations and doing whatever they wanted.

We have described above the contribution each developmental phase makes to the construction of a closed-system way of dealing with the challenges of adolescent development. To the contribution of cultural and peer variables we may add the vulnerability that results from earlier disruptions of attachment, problems of emotional attunement, a lack of parental availability, parental intrusiveness or indulgence, adult seductiveness, parental-child role reversals, and parental inability to provide containment. Experience with perverse power relations as a complex layering of multiple motives and functions derived from all levels of development confirms the perennial clinical experience of difficulty in working with patients who have found sadomasochistic ways to combat traumatic experiences of helplessness and thereby feel safe, good and effective.

TECHNICAL APPROACHES TO CLOSED-SYSTEM FUNCTIONING

Sadomasochism is a relational pathology and so will emerge in the treatment relationship from the very beginning. The adolescent has been functioning in a powerful, sadomasochistic way, probably for the whole of his or her life, and has practiced these styles of interacting with parents, teachers and peers. The patient's persistent search for pain or humiliation will be figured forth in the transference, often in subtle reactions to interpretations. The counter-reactions of the therapist may provide the first clue of underlying sadomasochistic functioning in the patient. The epigenetic layering of closed-system dynamics and their multiple functions emerge within the transference relationship and must be dealt with in that context.

The idea of two systems of conflict resolution and self-regulation can lead to a conceptualization of two kinds of technique, one that elucidates closed-system functioning, another that enhances open-system functioning. Conflicts over open-system functioning usually are expressed in reversion to closed-system omnipotent beliefs, efforts at creating sadomasochistic interactions and relationships, and externalization of impulses or ego and superego functions onto the analyst. Technical interventions have differing impacts on phenomena relating to the two systems. We need a broad spectrum of techniques to address closed-system functioning. We can now summarize what we have found useful and effective.

First is to *respect* the patient's closed system as a creative solution to a problem, not just as a problem to be eradicated. One major difference between our two-systems model of self-regulation and many other current approaches to affect regulation is their emphasis on *deficiencies* in "competent self-regulation." Whether the theory or technique emphasizes primary "Executive Function Disorder" (Palombo, 2011), or right brain dysfunctions related to attachment disorders (Schore, 2002), or inabilities to "mentalize" (Fonagy et al., 2002), or other theories of genetic anomalies or chemical imbalance, they all propose that maladaptive or pathological behavior stems from a lack or deficiency in affect- or self-regulatory capacity. In our view, whatever the cause, all people find a way to regulate their affects.

When we see a preschool child having a temper tantrum or hear that an adolescent gets into overwhelming rages that keep him up all night plotting revenge, or read about the Nobel Prize-winning author who feels driven to seduce every woman he meets, these all represent forms of self-regulation. We may think that they are pathological, but closed-system modes can be highly effective and powerful. Perversion works, up to a point. Verbalizing this often produces a profound feeling of being understood and a feeling of relief. As omnipotent beliefs emerge, we connect them to the underlying experience of helplessness. This points the way to finding alternative solutions.

One of the first interventions was to ask Nick how often he thinks of suicide, since most sadomasochistic patients have this in the background. He seemed relieved to talk of his frequent thoughts and plans to kill himself. He was going to use his mother's medication—he thought that this would be "ironic"; *she* would be responsible for *his* death. The story of his guilt and omnipotent responsibility for his mother's depression and breakdown unfolded. I empathized with his helplessness and acknowledged the idea of suicide as one solution. He expected me to try to talk him out of the idea of suicide, but I said that he would always have that as a solution and in fact it would end whatever problems he was having. I could hear how angry, desperate, and guilty he was feeling, but perhaps we could find alternative ways of dealing with the issues.

Next we can look together at *what needs are being met*—what problem is being solved by the closed-system response? This includes discovering the various functions being served by closed-system, hostile or submissive relationships, how the sadomasochism replaces superego controls of feelings and behavior, and the sources of instinctual gratification that are implicated.

We described earlier Nick's initial presentation as someone in pain and discomfort. He thought he was just being "weird," but from his mother's letter about his infancy we could see this as a way of being together. I said that everyone needs to feel attached to people, but we each find our own way. There is nothing weird in the need, but we can work to expand his ways to get together with others. This soon led to his closed-system overwhelming guilt. I said that everyone needs to have an internal compass and a signal of straying too far from the direction one sets. But his compass seems unrelated to "true North" and, instead of a signal, he gets a high voltage charge which is further disorienting. We then talked about everyone's need to protect themselves and how most of the "weird" things he described, such as his religious phase as a school child when he was sure that he would "burn in hell," his substance abuse in high school, and his current suicide wishes are all attempts to protect himself. The aim of our work, I said, was to increase his ways of self protection, so that he is not limited to attacking himself as the only solution. For Nick, suicide represented his ultimate omnipotent belief that he could change his mother, make her better, absolve himself and force her to be the mother he needed.

Then we listen for *omnipotent beliefs*, which can come in many forms and may or may not be conscious. Often the omnipotent belief that the patient's sadomasochism controls other people is conscious. Severe guilt or inhibition of action is often connected with a conscious belief in power to hurt and destroy others. Gentle reality confrontation, for example, "Has your experience with me so far indicated that I would be so angry that I would throw you out?" keeps the analyst in touch with actuality and offers the patient some contrast. Over time one effect of such interventions is to contribute to the necessary creation of conflict within the ego. With repeated shared experiences that magical beliefs don't change anything or anybody, especially the analyst, the focus can shift to exploring their sources, then seeking alternatives.

Much of the work with Nick uncovered omnipotent beliefs that were the major engine for his pathological behavior. He internalized the accusations of his brother and parents that he was responsible for upsetting those around him and even sending mother to hospital with a major biological depression. He ended up feeling special, super-powerful, and capable of driving anyone crazy. He felt so powerful that nothing could stop him except turning those powers against himself.

In his school years, he developed a beating fantasy as a way of controlling his omnipotent aggression. Nick's whole life could be seen as living out a beating fantasy, but sometime in later elementary school, he began to believe that he would be unjustly attacked. He imagined raising his hand with the answer in class and being shot down by the teacher and ridiculed by his classmates. His own anger and demeaning rage toward others were projected. In his brother and father he found obvious "validation" of his beating fantasy. Then he could feel justified in doing hostile and sadistic things to others.

This evolved into massive substance abuse in adolescence and then in late adolescence into suicidal fantasies and a major constriction of activity. Anything he did or accomplished had to be done in secret. He believed that his achievements would make others sick with envy and he would be responsible for their pain. His major defense, mode of attachment and sexual discharge was sadomasochistic with the omnipotent belief that he had found the magical solution to all his problems. These beliefs were linked to the reality of his helplessness as an infant, child, and adolescent.

Lastly, and very importantly, we look at the operation of *externalization* in all family members. Mutual externalizations and internalizations create a complex family system that requires careful analysis, with the interpersonal psychological exchanges detailed. Each step in the sequence carries and evokes different emotions. In describing the development of Nick's defensive omnipotence, we noted many instances where his parents' externalizations impacted his personality formation. Most centrally, they dealt with their own helplessness by externalizing responsibility onto Nick. This led to his internalizing the blame and generating an omnipotent belief that he was a monster. They also externalized their own experience of intense sibling hatred and rivalry on to the two boys, and dealt with their own guilt by normalizing it. Both boys took this in and recreated the scenario. Parent work focused on these issues, while the work with Nick also addressed the sequence of externalizing and internalizing defenses.

Externalization is a central mechanism in closed-system functioning. It represents a way of relating that is in itself abusive, as it violates the reality of the other (Novick, J. and Novick, K. K., 2007 [1994]). We describe this as based on "soul blindness," the inability or defensive refusal to see others as they really are (Wurmser, 1994; Novick, K. K and Novick, J., 2005). This is the antithesis of attunement. Omnipotence of thought or deed is a potential fantasy response to any experienced helplessness, but as a *fixed* delusional conviction in an adolescent it is usually embedded in a lifelong interaction with parents who deal with their own anxieties by the imposition of their omnipotent defenses in enactments with their children. Adolescent development poses threats to parental omnipotent defenses against their helplessness in the face of advancing years and accelerating decline and parents may react in various extreme ways. Parents of adolescents often suddenly seek divorce, have affairs, lose jobs, move precipitately, become seriously ill, any of which may serve to confirm the adolescent's sense of destructive omnipotent power.

Externalization is a broad category encompassing all the mental mechanisms of attributing the inside to the outside. We have distinguished among various forms of externalization, since they each respond to different interventions (Novick, J. and Novick, K. K., 2007 [1996]). Such mechanisms appear outside treatment, and, within the treatment relationship, in the form of an externalizing transference. Positive aspects of the patient's self, as well as negative ones, can be externalized on to the analyst.

In Nick's case the first type of externalization was of the helpless, confused, frustrated self of infancy described above. This is what is often called "projective identification," a term we find confusing and unhelpful as it condenses too many steps. Also, to privilege one's feelings as an indicator of the truth is an omnipotent move by the therapist. Therapists can instead use their own feelings as an initial signal and then wonder with the patient whether he was made to feel that way in his childhood, to find out together with the patient if this is an externalization of an earlier self-experience. In Nick's case, this technique was what led to the letter from his mother about his infancy.

Next to appear was the form of externalization we call "generalization," where the person assumes that others are like him. Nick thought that I was as competitive, hostile, critical and vulnerable as he was. So he had to avoid any action or thought that might lead to a major battle. The first intervention here is to appeal to his rational mind and ask if there is anything I had said or done to warrant such a view. We could then explore together where this type of shared hostility had actually occurred; this led us to the history of rivalrous, hostile competition with his brother and father. With this genetic material, transference aspects could safely be explored.

As we noted earlier, given the security and gratification that sadomasochistic functioning provide to the individual, it is questionable why anyone would give it up. What is the alternative? The patient fears that the only alternative is the primitive states of helplessness, rage or traumatic guilt that originally gave rise to the defensive omnipotent delusions of closed-system functioning.

To think about an alternative and techniques to support it that provide hope to both patient and therapist, we have to consider and reconsider some of our basic psychoanalytic assumptions. Psychoanalysis is, above all, a developmental theory and a model of development that informs all kinds of therapeutic techniques either implicitly or directly.

Freud described various developmental models, but the one that is most used, even clung to, by modern psychoanalysts of all schools, is what we term a "single-track" model (Novick, K. K. and Novick, J., 2002).

Other analytic writers before us have critiqued single-track developmental theory (Peterfreund, 1978; Silverman, 1981; Gillette, 1992). Their cogent arguments tend to be ignored, however, and there seems to be a perennial pull, both theoretically and clinically, for psychoanalysts to stress a unitary pathological continuum. Gabbard, a prominent, classically trained American psychoanalyst, cited Ferro, Ogden, and Bion to agree that "we oscillate between the depressive and the paranoid-schizoid throughout our lives" (2009, p. 586). This implies neglect of the individual's strengths, capacities and push toward progressive development, with underestimation of the opportunities provided by reality experience, including that of the treatment situation and relationship. Many of the findings of current observational and experimental infant research and of neurobiological studies confirm the existence of motivations and areas of functioning that are outside conflict, and imply motives of competence and mastery (Schore, 1994). There is no indication that normally endowed infants go through early phases of pathological functioning, only to emerge intact as normally functioning children. Equally, those individuals who suffer extreme hardship and deprivation in infancy do not uniformly develop later pathology; resiliency and self-righting demand explanation (Werner and Smith, 1982; Moskowitz, 1983; Anthony and Cohler, 1987; Kagan, 1996; Sroufe, 1996; Cicchetti and Nurcombe, 2007).

There is a fundamental need in everyone for homeostasis and mastery, which underlie a sense of self and self-esteem. Each person needs to feel safe, that his world is predictable, that his experience is encompassable, that obstacles can be overcome, problems can be solved and conflicts resolved. From infancy on, individuals can feel pleasure when such conditions can be assumed. In the closed system the basis for mastery and self-regulation is omnipotent belief in the power and necessity to be a perpetrator or victim in order to survive. In the open system the method of mastering inner and outer forces is the maximum use of one's genuine mental and physical capacities to be realistically effective and competent.

The closed and open systems do not differentiate people, that is, they are not diagnostic categories. Rather, the constructs describe potential choices of adaptation *within each individual at any challenging point in development* and allow for a metapsychological or multidimensional description of the components of the individual's relation to himself and others. Each of the metapsychological dimensions can fruitfully be applied to the two systems, as we have done in our discussions of love (Novick, J. and Novick, K. K., 2000) and the superego (Novick, J. and Novick, K. K., 2004). It should also be evident that the topographical point of view, delineating conscious, preconscious and unconscious content and functioning, applies equally to the open and closed systems.

We want to emphasize that everything we describe about working with open and closed systems in patients applies also to therapists and psychoanalysts. We all have a professional duty to monitor and differentiate open- and closed-system functioning in ourselves as well as in the patient. This helps us to stay grounded in the face of the inevitable pull to sadomasochistic enactments.

One way to characterize the goal of treatment is in terms of movement out of characteristic closed-system self-regulation to greater open-system functioning (Novick, J. and Novick, K. K., 2006). At the end of a good-enough treatment, the patient has not "grown beyond" closed-system modes of self-regulation but has developed the capacity to choose open-system solutions that have been nurtured and practiced in the therapeutic relationship. In our view, psychoanalysis has traditionally elaborated substantive understanding and treatment of closed-system pathology, but there has been insufficient attention to the co-existing operation of open-system capacities.

Earlier we described some of the work on elucidating and engaging with Nick's closed-system hostile omnipotent beliefs and how they functioned both to serve basic needs and fuel his pathology. We noted that these life-long, closed-system adaptations to trauma were effective and could not be set aside unless the patient experienced viable alternatives for meeting legitimate basic needs, such as defense against trauma, attachment and discharge. Technical interventions have differing impacts on phenomena relating to the two systems. Closed-system phenomena require the drive/defense, classical approach of transference and resistance analysis, with the aim of putting the patient in the active center of his pathology. But defense and transference interpretations of open-system functioning can pathologize and drive away competence. Mirroring, empathy, reconstruction, validation, support, and developmental education, to list but a few, link open-system phenomena with the therapist's functions beyond serving only as a transference object. These techniques applied to closed-system functioning, however, may be at best a palliative waste of time; at worst, they may serve to reinforce a passive, helpless, victimized stance on the part of the patient. Thus, we have to think in terms of expanded and alternative technical options to encompass the open-system dimensions of our patients' personalities and the opportunities of the treatment situation. This expansion encompasses reclaiming a broad spectrum of techniques and inclusion of work with parents of adolescent patients (Novick, K. K and Novick, J., 2002).

Initially the two systems are a theoretical heuristic device that exists mainly in the therapist's mind. The goal is to bring to the surface or to the foreground hidden, unacknowledged or potential open-system capacities. To illustrate some of the technical approaches that promote this process, we will describe more material through the phases of Nick's six-year psychoanalytic treatment and his return ten years after for brief further work.

TECHNIQUES FOR INCLUDING AND
FOSTERING THE OPEN SYSTEM

A major manifestation of open-system functioning in treatment is in the patient's and therapist's joint creation of a therapeutic alliance throughout. The therapeutic alliance concept functions as a lens that helps us focus on the capacities and motivations, conscious and unconscious, from all levels of the personality and all stages of development that enter into the collaborative tasks of each phase of treatment. The specific therapeutic alliance tasks of any particular phase of treatment confront resistances arising from closed-system functioning (Novick, K.K. and Novick, J., 1998), the major obstacle to developmental and therapeutic progression.

Simultaneously with the usual clinical work of listening, empathizing and engaging with Nick's closed-system pain, rage, and suicidal revenge, I also listened for and tried to engage with areas of open-system functioning. Sometimes this meant finding the positive aspect of what he presented as a confession of sadistic behavior. For example, he described how his older brother had slipped on the kitchen door threshold when stepping down into the garage. Nick, who was only in kindergarten then, immediately sized up the physical situation and pulled the kitchen door over his brother's legs trapping him and making him totally helpless. Brother and parents were in a rage and never let him forget how nasty he was. I took this as further evidence of how furious he was at his brother, but also commented on the high level spatial intelligence he displayed. "If I had been there," I said, "I might have said that kid is going to be an engineer one day!" which was indeed his first chosen profession.

There were other examples of high-level ego capacities being co-opted for sadistic purposes, like his teaching himself at age six to operate a reel-to-reel tape recorder, then hiding the recording device to tape the older brother's sadistic comments to both younger children when baby-sitting. I registered and later commented on his resourcefulness, his being extremely smart, his bravery and will to fight back and not just give up. I extended the evaluation so that I could look for open-system potential, feel some hope that our work together could bring significant change and get beyond his initial presentation as a weird, suicidal, inhibited, asocial character, and find something to like and admire.

The evaluation period was also a time to discern some internal conflicts and set therapeutic goals. The analyst as transference object is crucial for work on the closed system but, for open-system functioning, the analyst also has to set himself as a representative of reality, someone who has some ideas about past and current possibilities. This then includes setting, with the patient, some realistic goals for the treatment. In Nick's case I could comment on his history as presented by him and his parents as one of trauma, abuse and "soul blindness" by his parents. One result was that his extraordinary capacities were used in the service of protection and attack, and they were seen by all, including him, as weapons of mass destruction. He was inhibiting his creativity, doing things in secret and getting no joy in being so naturally talented. He only got secret triumphant pleasure in beating others. One of our goals could be to help him find pride and pleasure in his capacities and creativity.

Nick's parents were an integral part of his treatment from the beginning. Although that is not the focus of this contribution, it is important to state that regular concurrent parent work throughout elucidated the history, inter-generational dynamics and possibilities for change. We have written elsewhere about the significant role of parent work in treatments for children and adolescents (Novick, K. K. and Novick, J., 2005, 2009).

Mastery of alliance tasks and internalization of the therapeutic alliance build on and promote open-system consolidation. Children, adolescents and adults finish good-enough treatment with the potential for adaptive transformations in response to the many challenges of life (Novick, J. and Novick, K. K., 2006, 2009). These begin in the evaluation phase of treatment, when the analyst works to initiate transformations of self-help to joint work; chaos to order and meaning; fantasies to realistic goals; external complaints and circumstantial explanations to internal meanings, motivations and conflicts; helplessness to competence; despair to hopefulness.

The early months of Nick's treatment were spent, as we described earlier, with both patient and analyst in discomfort. He could not lie on the couch for fear I would attack him and could not bear to sit in the chair opposite for fear I would see his critical, sadistic thoughts. We eventually settled on his sitting behind me. Much work was done via the transference to me of feelings and beliefs related to his parents and his brother. We could verbalize his conviction that he was a monster able to drive his brother crazy, intensify father's competitiveness and send mother to hospital. This helped, but a major shift occurred when I took up the reality that I had actually allowed him to sit behind me. I knew that he had critical, hostile, even sadistic thoughts about me, but I trusted that he also had enough good feelings inside and enough "emotional muscle" to control himself and not put his feelings into action. He was no longer a child and knew the difference between feelings and actions.

As an athletic young man, the idea of "emotional muscle" intrigued him. This ushered in a period of describing and working on building the emotional muscle to regulate his feelings; to accept the idea that he is in charge of himself but cannot force the reactions of others; to know what he was actually in control of and what he was helpless to change, for instance, the envious reactions of others. This led back to his wish to be all-powerful, to be the one responsible for the envy of others. He was beginning to experience an internal conflict between his wish to be magically omnipotent, in charge of everything and everybody, on the one hand, and, on the other, to enjoy the possibilities of reality and accept the limits of his power and responsibility. One day, as he sat behind me, I could hear restless movements. I asked what he was doing and he said, "I think that I'm pumping myself up so that I can have the emotional muscle to know my feelings won't destroy you and make you attack me. I want to be strong enough to be able to sit in front of you and let you look at me."

From the alliance task of *being with,* highlighted in the beginning phase of treatment, can come confidence in the capacity to be alone with oneself, to value oneself and to cooperate in a trusting, mutually enhancing relationship with others. The analyst's therapeutic alliance task in this phase is to *feel with* the patient. Empathy and modeling true interest and enjoyment become important factors to counter externalizations and skewed relationships of dominance and submission.

The task of *working together* in the middle phase challenged Nick's omnipotent belief that others would be beaten, threatened or destroyed by his achievements. His protection was to do things alone and in secret. As the work progressed I commented on the times we worked well, when together we accomplished more than either alone. I pointed out the reality that his good work did not threaten or hurt me, and, most importantly, noted explicitly when the work together was pleasurable. Initially those open-system moments were almost non-existent or were so fleeting that they could easily pass unremarked. When we spotted the operation of an omnipotent belief, we traced it developmentally, reconstructing each phase in the evolution of his closed-system responses. This process brings the underlying magical assumptions into secondary process consideration to be explored.

"Developmental images" are often effective and unthreatening tools for this effort (Novick, J. and Novick, K. K., 2003). These provide a safely displaced, neutral context in which the patient can feel understood and can experience the analyst's empathy as a contrast to the emotionally absent parent. Here the analyst is a teacher who has the knowledge and experience to speak with authority. For example, I described how all toddlers generalize the behavior of their own parents to all other adults. So if parents react negatively to a certain type of behavior, the toddler believes that everyone else will too. That makes it hard for him to credit his own experience and trust other grownups.

Noting the pleasure of cooperative work led to Nick's obvious anxiety in feeling good. He would slip back into silence or inhibition; we could then focus on his conflict over ordinary good feelings. This was a new conflict, one clearly between closed-system sadistic triumph and open-system mutual pleasure. "This is nuts" he said, "feeling good makes me feel scared!" It also made him feel lonely and sad, realizing how much he missed not having anyone to share things with. This work led to his willingness to take an opportunity to cooperate with a retired scientist. Together they created an innovative and still much-used virtual computer program. "I guess Prof. is the father I never had. I still find myself thinking he'll be upset at something I figure out but in fact he's delighted. It's like you said, most people enjoy doing things together."

We did extensive work on Nick's rage at women and his omnipotent defenses against feeling helpless to get what he needed from his mother. It is clinically important to acknowledge and verbalize the intense experience of anger. We address this as an unfinished task from toddlerhood, when parents should ordinarily help the child master feelings and transform feeling-states into useful signal affect. Adolescent patients like Nick respond well to reconstruction of this failure in early interactions, recognizing the dynamic and often feeling strong empathy and sympathy for their younger selves.

This work had enabled him to start going out with women, but he always managed to do something to have them disappoint him; then he could reject them. Here was a later version of his school-aged beating fantasy. He provoked a hostile attack, believed himself to be an innocent victim, and then could neglect the woman without guilt. Nick felt relieved when each relationship ended. We talked about his belief that he had to be invulnerable, never to be surprised by a rejection. He could always be in charge and make it happen. I agreed that being alone is a powerful protection, but then reminded him of the pleasure he had in doing things together. Perhaps he could work to build up the emotional muscle to tolerate rejection. We could use the experiences of separation in our relationship to exercise those muscles and practice making distinctions among rejections, losses and ordinary absences. Some time later Nick had a relationship that ended when the woman went back to her old boyfriend. "It is sad, I feel hurt," he said, "but it's not the end of the world. I'm still me and I'll keep going. I don't quit when I lose a tennis match, why should I quit going out. It's better than convincing myself that I don't need anyone but really being very lonely."

The new level and range of ego functions used to *work together* in alliance with the analyst throughout the middle of analysis can be used for living and for self-analysis. In addition to ego functions such as memory, perception, self-reflection, integration, and so forth are the metacognitive functions that Freud referred to as the executive function of the ego, and that Anna Freud described as the general characteristics of the personality. Included here would be the capacity to plan, anticipate, work through a task from beginning to completion, take pleasure in the process and so forth. We have described these as "emotional muscles" developed throughout life with support from parents and community;

they play a crucial role in determining health, creativity and resilience (Novick, K. K and Novick, J., 2010, 2011).

As the patient becomes aware that there are other and more sustainable ways to maintain safety and good feelings, an *internal conflict* develops between the two modes of self-regulation, the old, closed omnipotent system and the newly-rediscovered system of open, competent functioning. With this internal change, there is increased motivation for progression and additional leverage to address the range of pathology, with its underpinnings of clinging to omnipotent beliefs. The interrelationship of closed-system superego pathology and sadomasochism is central to the work with many such patients, as it was with Nick, who used his beating fantasy instead of a functioning superego (Novick, J. and Novick, K. K., 1972, 2005b, 2007 [1996]). Wurmser's extensive work on "vicious cycles" and the harsh "inner judge" is particularly illuminating in regard to the way sadomasochism functions in lieu of a superego to undermine clinical progress in the context of the therapeutic relationship (2007). Nick's fierce inhibition of functioning denoted a struggle between his belief in his own omnipotent power to destroy and his wish/fear that no one else could control him.

The conscious experience of conflict between open- and closed-system ways of functioning puts pressure on the treatment. Emerging satisfaction, creative joy, and objective love for the self and the other threaten old closed-system patterns of defense against helplessness, trauma, anxiety, guilt and depression. Just as we saw how pain is used to maintain the closed system, so pleasure is the motivation and reinforcer of the open system. When significant changes begin to occur in treatment, the resistances often focus on the danger of pleasure and the threat this poses to the closed system. There is a strong pull to stay with the familiar closed-system belief that everything can be controlled if pleasure is restricted and avoided.

The arena for understanding, change, and growth in treatment and beyond is the therapeutic relationship. Often the transference aspects of the relationship lend themselves most to elucidating closed-system phenomena. Open-system functioning unfolds in the relationship context of the therapeutic alliance and the use of the analyst as a developmental object, who stands for reality and offers authoritative knowledge and experience for both modeling and identification. Open-system technique pays explicit attention to good ego functioning, to the pleasure inherent in using physical, intellectual, social and emotional skills effectively (*funktionslust*), noting when capacities are not accessible or brought constructively into action. The two-systems model reclaims analytic legitimacy for prematurely discarded supportive and psycho-educational techniques as integral to therapeutic work.

Nick graduated from university, worked for a few years, met a woman he wanted to marry and said that he thought he was ready to end his analysis soon. He called his closed system "my crap magic program or MCMP." "It's still there," he said, "especially when I get pissed at my girlfriend, but then I realize I have alternatives to destroying our relationship. I can talk to her and that usually works. And if it doesn't, I'm OK; I can stand being angry for a while without everything collapsing." He went on, "I'm glad that you said that MCMP never goes away or I would be thinking that I'm a failure or you're a failure. I realize that our work together has given me choices and most of the time I can set my crap system aside and enjoy reality. I can still get a moment's high thinking of how I can drive my brother green with envy. But it doesn't last or get me anywhere. My ordinary pleasures of work and my friends are really much more satisfying and dependable."

We have emphasized the omnipotent, sadomasochistic solution as a defense that people will do anything to protect, including self-injury or suicide. Patients have little incentive to change the adaptations they have clung to, perhaps from earliest childhood. They do not come into treatment to have their sadomasochistic solutions eradicated or taken away — in fact, they worry that this might be the analyst's goal, in collusion with spouses, parents, employers, courts and other authority figures. They usually accept help because omnipotent solutions are not working well enough and then try to cast the therapist as another omnipotent figure they can control by sadomasochistic means. Treatment will not eradicate pathological, closed-system solutions. Rather we work to create a safe setting in which the patient can experiment with alternative open-system solutions, with the knowledge that sadomasochism is never sublimated, relinquished, demolished, resolved, but only set aside when more adaptive and fulfilling solutions are available.

Open-system use of ego functions is consolidated in the *independent therapeutic work* begun during pretermination, then continued after treatment whenever necessary. Other dimensions of ego growth are resilience and creativity. The emotional muscles needed to tolerate frustration, encompass failure, integrate disappointment and disparity realistically, and register pleasure and mastery contribute to increasing access to creativity in all realms of life. Technically, these open-system manifestations have to be explicitly named, acknowledged and consolidated for successful treatment and growth.

When the patient falters and ego functioning dips, the analyst can check whether the patient notices and address the conflicts over independent perception and responsibility. This was an ongoing task, but, at this time in the treatment, I noticed that I was doing more work than usual. Nick couldn't remember his past sessions, associate or engage in exploring his fantasies. One clue was my feeling that I was particularly effective. I then asked Nick if he noticed that he seemed unable to do the work. I wondered if it had anything to do with our relationship. I shared my feeling about being especially clever and wondered if he might be shutting down in some way to make me feel good.

This appeared to turn things around. Nick linked his behavior in the sessions with his remarkable success on a new project at work. He was afraid that I would feel diminished and envious. Nick's closed-system fear that his success would destroy his parents and brother re-emerged. But more central at this point was the priority of developing the muscle to hold on to and tolerate the reality that he was actually happier and more emotionally successful than the rest of his family.

A good goodbye to treatment depends on the patient's, the analyst's and the parents' capacities to bear feelings, mourn losses and internalize good aspects of the other. Each of the therapeutic alliance tasks for patient, therapist and parents or significant others is a manifestation or objective description of an aspect of the open system. Such a conceptualization helps us maintain criteria internal to the clinical situation for the assessment of obstacles, change and eventual termination. Mastery and internalization of the therapeutic alliance tasks propel the patient and his parents through the treatment trajectory to reach the dual goals of restoration to progressive development and transformation of the parent-child relationship. At termination Nick faced and experienced his sadness—his emotional muscles had been strengthened by the work of his analysis.

Sadness is part of the open system; one is sad only about leaving something one loves. Nick and I could both experience and express our sadness as the treatment ended. He contrasted the sadness he was feeling with the emptiness he felt throughout his childhood and adolescence. "That was truly unbearable and no wonder I needed weed and booze to get me through each day. This is different. I feel very sad but not empty. I feel full of all kinds of good stuff. This is a very special relationship where you give me your full attention for this whole hour. But I'm OK and I know that I can come back if I need to."

"Wait! If I *want* to."

I received a letter two years later telling me that he had married the woman he had dated at the end of our work and that he now had a child. Nick wrote, "I remember telling you that I would never be stupid enough to love anyone. Well, that was my crap magic program talking. I'm hopelessly, helplessly and completely in love with my little fellow and I feel that I've really pushed MCMP aside and I've grown up."

Nick resumed treatment briefly ten years later via Skype, phone, and visits. His wife was having serious psychological difficulties and he first called for a referral. She was diagnosed with depression that didn't seem to respond to medication. She was reluctant to start a psychoanalytic treatment and Nick was feeling frustrated, helpless, frightened, and angry. When he called, he said he needed help because he found himself constantly thinking of running away. He said the only thing that stopped him was his love for his son, who needed him to be there for him and his mother. Nick did not want his boy to feel what he had felt growing up. Ten years earlier, having set aside his closed omnipotent system, Nick was able to opt primarily for open-system modes of self-regulation and move into a joyful, loving and creative adulthood. In his second, briefer period of treatment Nick used his capacities to think through clearly what his choices could be and determine a constructive and satisfying life path.

Life is not easy; there are no guarantees, but Nick's analysis equipped him with open-system tools to engage with the inevitable difficulties of life. Expansion and strengthening of ego functions and emotional muscles throughout treatment are at the center of our understanding of therapy as a developmental experience. Strengthening the open system of self-regulation helps to equalize the forces in the life-long struggle against the developmentally determined and culturally reinforced hostile, omnipotent, sadomasochistic power dynamics of the closed system.

NOTE

1. In this chapter we have chosen to use "I" when referring to the analyst in actual clinical interactions, and the collective "we/our/us" when describing our joint, general theoretical, technical and clinical formulations. The "I" is an attempt to capture some of the immediacy of the work and it also adds another layer of confidentiality to the reported clinical material.

REFERENCES

Anthony, J., and Cohler, B. (1987). *The Invulnerable Child*. New York and London: Guilford.

Blum, H. (1980). Paranoia and beating fantasy: An inquiry into the psychoanalytic theory of paranoia. *Journal of the American Psychoanalytic Association* 28: 331–62.

Cichetti, D., and Nurcombe, B. (2007). The long-term consequences of childhood emotional maltreatment on development: (Mal)adaptation in adolescence and young adulthood. *Child Abuse & Neglect* 33: 19–21.

Cicchetti, D., and Rogosch, F. (1996). Equifinality and multifinality in developmental psychopathology. *Development and Psychopathology* 8: 597–600.

DeVito, E. (2009). Attachment relationships from adolescence to adulthood. Paper presented at conference of Munich Association for Psychoanalysis, November 2009.

Doidge, N. (2007). *The Brain That Changes Itself*. New York: Viking Press.

Fonagy, P., Gergely, G., Jurist, E., and Target, M. (2002). *Affect Regulation, Mentalization, and the Development of Self*. New York: Other Press.

Freud, S. (1916). Some character-types met with in psychoanalytic work. *Standard Edition* 14: 311–36.

Gabbard, G. (2009). What is a "good enough" termination? *Journal of the American Psychoanalytic Association* 57: 575–94.

Gillette, E. (1992). Psychoanalysts' resistance to new ideas. *Journal of the American Psychoanalytic Association* 40: 1232–35.

Kagan, J. (1996). Three pleasing ideas. *American Psychologist* 51: 901–7.

Moskowitz, S. (1983). *Love Despite Hate*. New York: Schocken.

Novick, J., and Novick, K. K. (1972). Beating fantasies in children. *International Journal of Psychoanalysis* 70: 237–42.

——— (2000). Love in the therapeutic alliance. *Journal of the American Psychoanalytic Association* 48: 189-218.

——— (2001). Two systems of self-regulation. *Journal of Psychoanalytic Social Work* 8: 95–122.

——— (2003). Two systems of self-regulation and the differential application of psychoanalytic technique. *American Journal of Psychoanalysis* 63: 1–19.

——— (2004). The superego and the two-systems model. *Psychoanalytic Inquiry* 24: 232–56.

——— (2005a). Soul blindness: A child must be seen to be heard. In *Divorce and Custody: Contemporary Developmental Psychoanalytic Perspectives*, eds. L. Gunsberg and P. Hymowitz. Washington, D.C.: American Psychological Association Books, 81–90

——— (2005b). The superego and the two-system model. *Psychoanalytic Inquiry* 24: 232–56.

——— (2006). *Good Goodbyes: Knowing How to End in Psychotherapy and Psychoanalysis.* New York: Jason Aronson.

——— (2007 [1994]). Externalization as a pathological form of relating: the dynamic underpinnings of abuse. In *Fearful Symmetry: The Development And Treatment Of Sadomasochism*. Northvale, NJ: Jason Aronson, 147–70.

——— (2007 [1996]). *Fearful Symmetry: The Development And Treatment Of Sadomasochism.* Northvale, NJ: Jason Aronson.

——— (2009). The Rat Man and two systems of self-regulation. Round Robin Newsletter. *American Psychological Association Division of Psychoanalysis* 24(1): 1, 11–17.

——— (In press). A new model of techniques for concurrent psychodynamic work with parents of child and adolescent psychotherapy patients. In *Psychodynamic Psychotherapy*, eds. R. Ritvo and S. Papilsky, Child and Adolescent Psychiatric Clinics of North America.

Novick, K. K., and Novick, J. (1987). The essence of masochism. *Psychoanalytic Study of the Child* 42: 353–84.

——— (1998). An application of the concept of the therapeutic alliance to sadomasochistic pathology. *Journal of the American Psychoanalytic Association* 46: 813–46.

——— (2002). Reclaiming the land. *Psychoanalytic Psychology* 19: 348–77.

——— (2005). *Working With Parents Makes Therapy Work*. New York: Jason Aronson.

——— (2010). *Emotional Muscle: Strong Parents, Strong Children*. Indiana: XLibris.

——— (2011). Building emotional muscle in children and parents. *Psychoanalytic Study of the Child* 65: 131–51.

——— (In press). Exploring parent work in the treatment of late adolescents. In *Psychoanalytic Study of the Child*.

Palombo, J. (2011). Executive function conditions and self-deficits. In *Mental Health and Social Problems: A Social Work Perspective*, eds. N. Heller and A. Gitterman. New York: Routledge.

Peterfreund, E. (1978). Some critical comments on psychoanalytic conceptualizations in infancy. *International Journal of Psychoanalysis* 59: 427–41.

Sandler, J. and Freud, A. (1983). Discussions with Anna Freud on the ego and the mechanisms of defense: The ego and the id at puberty. *International Journal of Psychoanalysis* 64: 401–6.

Schore, A. N. (1994). *Affect Regulation and the Origins of the Self: The Neurobiology of Emotional Development*. Hillsdale, NJ: Lawrence Erlbaum.

——— (2002). Advances in neuropsychoanalysis, attachment theory, and trauma research: Implications for self psychology. *Psychoanalytic Inquiry* 22: 433–84.

Silverman, D. K. (1981). Some proposed modifications of psychoanalytic theories of early childhood development. In *Empirical Studies of Psychoanalytic Theories, Vol. 2*, ed. J. Maslin. Hillsdale, NJ: Analytic Press, 49–71.

Sroufe, L. A. (1996). *Emotional Development*. New York: Cambridge University Press.

Stern, D. (1985). *The Interpersonal World of the Infant*. New York: Basic Books.

Werner, E. E., and Smith, R. S. (1982). *Vulnerable But Invincible: A Longitudinal Study of Resilient Children and Youth*. New York: McGraw Hill.

Wurmser, L. (1994). A time of questioning: The severely disturbed patient within classical analysis. *The Annual of Psychoanalysis*, ed. J. A. Winer. Chicago Institute for Psychoanalysis, 173–207.

———— (1996). Trauma, inner conflict, and the vicious cycles of repetition. *Scandinavian Psychoanalytic Review* 19: 17–45.

———— (2007). *Torment Me, But Don't Abandon Me: Psychoanalysis of the Severe Neuroses in a New Key*. Lanham, MD: Rowman & Littlefield.

FOUR

Clinical Observations on Masochistic Character Structure

Robert Alan Glick, MD

I have found clinical work with masochistic character structure an absorbing and troubling challenge to psychoanalytic understanding and therapeutic effectiveness. In this chapter, I will describe those dynamic constructs I have found particularly useful in treating patients with masochistic features, and then offer clinical illustrations to describe certain technical challenges masochistic phenomena present in analytic treatments. These include examples of transference resistances and countertransference reactions that can dominate and paralyze these unsettling treatments.

My discussion will not address explicit sexual masochism, which, while involving pain, humiliation, subjugation, and powerlessness as features of overt sexual activity, is best considered from a separate clinical perspective and is beyond the scope of this chapter.

While it is a truism that pain and suffering are inescapable in life, interwoven with our common experiences of disappointment, failure, regret, loss, grief, shame and guilt, the driven pursuit of misery in masochism requires a complex and more disquieting understanding of mental life.

Clinical experience makes clear that all our patients come to us because they suffer. We assume that in crucial ways they cause their own pain and suffering in an effort to craft some unconscious compromise, to preserve or protect some unconscious wish or object or defend against greater pain. For Schafer (1988), perhaps all of our patients are masochistic to some degree:

[E]very disorder we work with clinically has its share of unhappiness and unfulfillment, and every one is characterized by repetitiousness, unconsciously designed and executed self injuriousness. Consequently, analysands seem to be bringing on much of the misery and need to do so. (p.88)

When the need to bring on misery dominates the clinical picture, when we suspect that the pursuit of suffering is a major organizing unconscious motivation, we face a grim test. It should be noted that this may be far from obvious in the initial presentation and assessment. Since our fundamental task is to understand and help ameliorate the sufferings of others, masochism unnerves us, troubles our sleep, causes us pain, and tests our strength. Nothing wounds us more than experiencing our well-intended therapeutic efforts as causing more pain and suffering. Consequently, we face particular obstacles and countertransference dilemmas in working with masochistic patients.

Masochism, defined as the motivated pursuit of pain and suffering, has been a theoretical and clinical challenge to psychoanalysis from its creation. In *Masochism: Current Psychoanalytic Perspectives*, Glick and Meyers introduced a collection of essays on the evolving psychoanalytic theoretical approaches to masochism, stating:

Just as psychoanalytic interest in masochism dates from the earliest days of psychoanalysis, the various approaches to its understanding have reflected the developmental vicissitudes of psychoanalytic theory as it moved from its earliest focus on instinct to considerations of psychic structure and oedipal dynamics, object relations, separation-individuation, self-organization, and self-esteem regulation, and as it progressed into more systematic investigation of child development. (1988, p. 1)

In that historical overview, we trace the emergence of psychoanalytic interest in sexual and characterological masochism to the publication in 1870 of Leopold von Sacher-Masoch's novel *Venus in Furs*. The novel portrays a male lover's passionate submission to forms of enslavement, failure, deprivation, humiliation, cruelty, and physical and psychological abuse for the sake of "love" and "sexual" pleasure. Interestingly, Sacher-Masoch alludes to many other dimensions and meanings in masochism: the role of the pre-oedipal, phallic mother, maternal loss, and narcissism.

The formal scientific examination of masochism as a sexual anomaly appeared in Kraft-Ebing's 1906 encyclopedic text *Psychopathica Sexualis*. Kraft-Ebing attributes the wish for pain, humiliation, and abuse to a congenital disorder of sexual instincts, equating passivity and femininity, as Freud problematically did.

Freud (1905) took up the issue early in the development of his psychosexual instinct theory, and he wrestled with it throughout his career in a series of papers, coining the term moral masochism (1924) to describe the need for punishment. Subsequently, psychoanalysts of various stripes have sought to fit masochism into their explanatory theories of mind and in their treatments.[1]

THEORETICAL ISSUES

Essentially, psychoanalysts seek to understand the nature of the unconscious desire, the driving fantasy or fantasies that the patient is attempting to gratify or recreate in their pursuit of pain and suffering.

Is the unrelenting pursuit of misery the product of a particular form of developmental trauma, the result of punitive or neglectful, subjugating or humiliating caregivers? Or does it reflect a particular temperamental vulnerability or failure of resilience of ego structures and self-organization?

For the analyst, there is no escaping the patient's insistence on suffering. Our major challenge is recognizing how, as we attempt to understand and help, we are drawn into becoming the agent of the patient's pain, the inevitable traumatizing, pathological object relation come alive in the transference.

I have wondered: Is a "successful" treatment of a person with significant masochism necessarily a painfully protracted reparative developmental process involving forms of mutual pain and suffering? Must the clinician be prepared to live with frustration and failure as the process moves slowly forward? And what defines a "successful" analytic treatment? Are we left with Freud's grim outcome goal of "everyday unhappiness?"

Theoretical Perspectives

In the clinical situation, the patient with masochistic character structure confronts us, broadly speaking, with his chronically punishing fate, life's unfairness, the selfishness and thoughtlessness of others and the conviction that nothing can or will ever change his tragic and miserable circumstances. Victimhood, asceticism and self-sacrifice are the only options. Pleasure remains elusive at best, and at worst an illusion, certainly for him. All efforts to change his mind, to show him his role in his suffering, only confirm his failure and defect.

As we become part of the patient's life, we are pulled into his unconscious world. We join in the misery as we come to experience periods, by turns fleeting and protracted, of despair, disappointment and defeat as our best efforts seem only to bring further suffering and victimization. In our countertransference reactions, we can become frustrated, angry and sadistic. We may wish to punish, humiliate, and abandon our patient, and thus confirm the patient's expectations.

My Guiding Dynamic Constructs

Nothing reveals the power of psychic reality over external reality more than masochism! Forget this at our peril; the patients know themselves most deeply through their self-defining attachment to their pain-inducing defenses.

Three interwoven core dynamic constructs help guide me in my clinical work:

1. The most familiar understanding of masochism rests on the role of unconscious guilt and harshness of superego punishment. We assume unconscious morality plays a central role in the structure of most neurotic, non-narcissistic, oedipal level conflict and becomes the focus of much of the analytic work. Interestingly, in training analyses, one can see masochistic submission in the form of the candidate's defensive idealization of the training analyst or the analysis. This serves as a tenacious resistance to fears of aggressive competitiveness. However, in general, in my experience, an oedipally based, superego punishment model is ineffective for more entrenched and severe masochistic character structure. I have found that an appreciation of narcissistic structures to be an important advance in our understanding.

2. Cooper's (1988) discussion of the relationship of masochism and narcissism opens an invaluable, deeper and ultimately more analytically effective understanding of masochism as a predominant character quality. Cooper defined the narcissistic-masochistic character structure (Glick and Meyers, 1988, pp.117–38) as based on the core defense of omnipotent control against unconsciously feared catastrophic trauma to the self from helplessness, humiliation, overwhelming envy and dissolution—a form of turning passive to active, of crafting a sense of agency. This is a significant shift away from the centrality of the Oedipus complex as the source of neurosis and move to self-esteem regulation, separation-individuation and early object relations as part of understanding masochism. In this model, the capacity for mature empathy (for self and others), tolerance of ambiguity and adaptive compromise is profoundly limited. All relationships, including necessarily the analytic relationship, suffer idealizations and devaluations, precipitous ruptures and tortured repairs. The capacity for genuine intimacy and love is a distant therapeutic and existential goal. However, I have found that masochistic pathology requires serious attention to the role of developmental trauma.

3. For individuals with a history of early and sustained developmental trauma, I have found it crucial to understand and respect the tenacity of the unconscious attachment to damaging and damaged,

selfish and cruel, fragile and demanding primary, usually severely narcissistic objects. Issues of boundaries, identity and impulse control shape their lives. These apparently wretched early relationships remain essential to maintaining self-cohesion and self-regulation. As a consequence, the patient develops complex identifications with the suffering of the primary objects—"keeping them alive through suffering." These are amongst the most persistent and severe forms of masochistic phenomena that I have encountered and therefore are often the heart-breaking and challenging treatments. The process of "transplanting" one pathological attachment with a new, analytic attachment can be interminable.

CLINICAL ILLUSTRATIONS OF VARIOUS MASOCHISTIC PHENOMENA

Lateness as an Example of a Sadomasochistic Homoerotic Narcissistic Transference

A patient in analysis whose chronic lateness is unmodified by the expectable interpretive efforts feels manifestly ashamed and guilty for this "bad behavior" which he labels masochistic. All explorations of rage, desire for punishment, implicit sexualized seduction, defiance and affect control produce deepening countertransference awareness of my being powerless to change this behavior and of being controlled.

Over time, the analysis reveals an unrelenting and sexually sadomasochistic attachment to a seductive, narcissistic, and absent parent. The patient's unconscious life has been consumed with displaced efforts to control the anxiety, the rage and the lustful desire for this powerful and elusive object.

As the lateness grew acutely worse, the patient complained of how painfully mortified he feels being so late, and yet he cannot stop himself. As we explored his mortification, he revealed that an upcoming event that represented a major and deeply hoped-for personal achievement would evoke excruciating guilt and intolerably dangerous envy in those he left behind. He dare not let his guard down and relax. He recognized that he had to exercise omnipotent control and self-punishment to balance what he was going to enjoy.

It hit me that I was what the patient was secretly treasuring; that of all the many meanings of his lateness, the most potent was how he used the humiliating lateness as a crucial expression of his omnipotent control. He wanted to keep the painful analysis going at a slow and tolerable pace and keep me in his life for as long as possible, as a (unacknowledgeable) replacement for a rejecting object choice.

Two Brief Examples of Seemingly Intractable Masochistic Character Pathology:
Neither in Analysis, Both in Forms of Explorative Psychotherapy

A Failed Treatment as an Example of Severe, Rigid Narcissistic Structure

A single businessman in his mid-forties entered psychotherapy with me after leaving a failed attempt at an analysis. He had had several prior treatments, always complaining of a lifetime of disappointment and a sense of lack of engagement in his life. He described a series of relationships with women to whom he feels obligated and not committed, and with whom he does not feel in love. He lacked real success in his work despite high intelligence and diligence. He came because he wanted relief from his chronic anxiety, pervasive despair, and sense of detachment and emptiness in his life.

We worked together in psychotherapy because he had lost faith in a deeper and more demanding treatment. I felt we had a good connection. He had a sense of humor which I realized gave me hope. We considered medication to relieve some of his anxiety and depression, which he accepted, and the largely supportive treatment began.

Early on, he brightened, made some changes, struggled to feel more involved. Ultimately, despite or perhaps because of my own active and engaged sense in the process, he sadly and bitterly confronted me with his feeling that I was not taking him and the problems seriously. I thought that this transference experience might allow him to explore the underlying narcissistic vulnerability and his defensive sense of devaluation. I tried to consider this with him. But he only took this as painful criticism. He felt very discouraged, so we mutually decided to stop, and he could call me to discuss further options. After one year went by, and he called, we met a couple of times. He was doing well at a job that paid inadequately to afford private treatment. I offered a reduced fee (my masochism?) or offered to refer him to our low cost psychoanalytic clinic. I have not heard back from him as yet.

The Need to Suffer as the Price of Pleasure

A married businessman in his mid-forties came to treatment because he has felt guilty and quietly depressed most of his life. He loves his wife and children and has a lovely, comfortable life. He seemed to have an obsessional character structure with depressive and masochistic features. Resisting an analysis for "practical" reasons and implicitly afraid of "opening up," he entered a psychotherapy with me, slowly did better, became less obsessed with guilt and punitive fantasies, but remained miserable in his work life and unable to find or risk a change. An antidepressant had helped some.

He seemed immovably stuck in his passivity, victimhood, feeling both lucky and shortchanged in life. Then, maybe as a result of the treatment and maybe not, he fell passionately in love with a woman with whom he works, a relationship he had never expected to find. He knew that he could not hurt his wife and children by leaving them. But he could not give up his lover who understands him deeply, with whom he feels unique passion and deep intimacy.

Tellingly, both he and his lover grew up in deeply compromised families dominated by physically and emotionally handicapped family members. For him, they had both been oppressed by a tragic fate. In a way that he felt he could not share with his happy wife, he felt he had found a soulmate.

For over three years of this parallel life, he lived in unremitting guilty fear of getting caught. He was both happier and more miserable than before. He focused on "being a bad person" because of this affair. As we continued to chip away at his dilemma of intractable guilty pleasure, the romance began to fade, and the passion cooled. He began to accept that they were not soul mates, and that he could envision "moving on" and making the best of his family life.

Interestingly, both these men had significant developmental traumas—the first with a psychotic father and volatile, difficult mother and two sisters whose lives are worse than his; the second with two developmentally severely damaged older brothers who completely dominated his family and caused him deep shame and guilt. The first has felt like trying to squirm out of heavy chains, and the second like swimming ever so slowing in thick mud.

An Extended Psychoanalysis Illustrating a Sadomasochistic Attachment

The following extended clinical illustration is a condensed account of a lengthy and deeply engaged fifteen-year analysis which ended several years ago. This is the story of the power of developmental trauma and the unfolding of a complex sadomasochistic attachment to an abusive, seductive and sadly needy, "soul murdering" (the patient's term from his reading of the Shengold book) mother. From him and this treatment, I learned about the profound, tenacious and unconscious power of this complex, miserable bond as the analysis slowly proceeded to reveal his tragic internal world.

The patient had come to see me after college graduation. He was depressed, anxious, immobilized, and lost about what direction to take and feeling trapped in an emotional bunker living with his mother. His mother had exercised control over most aspects of his life including his choice of analyst. Her particular concern was whether I could teach how to be what she considered a responsible adult in the world, especially in dealing with money. This issue would come to have many painful and fantastic meanings over the years.

His family was wealthy and socially prominent. When he was around nine, his parents went through what he recalled as a "bloody" divorce. There had been much battling and belittling of each other. The father was the target of family denigration.

The patient grew up feeling very protective of his younger sibling, especially as the horrific picture of his life emerged in the analysis. This violent and tumultuous divorce was the beginning of the end of any sense of a loving and realistically validating family life.

In the beginning of the analysis, the work focused on helping him understand why he felt so inadequate, so stuck both at home and in a failed relationship with a girlfriend he rarely saw and who cheated on him. While very polite and pseudo-compliant, he gradually revealed that he feared I was basically an agent of his mother. Since she was grudgingly paying the bill, he assumed that I might actually be reporting back to her about his progress in the treatment. He was not delusional because the mother had indeed exerted control over most aspects of his life and may have ended a prior treatment. Very slowly, he could acknowledge why he had needed to maintain this idea of my role as his mother's agent. In this way, he could hold on to her and at the same time attempt to free himself from her grip. His father had selfishly left him to suffer with her and was judged a tragic failure for the patient. It was difficult to imagine what role I could play in his emotional life.

The early transference was superficially idealizing but fearful and masochistic (and quietly paranoid). He would submit to me but not really trust me. He had both a timid, submissive, and a haughty disregard for the treatment frame, being late, missing sessions and leaving bills unpaid for a couple of months or more.

What impressed me early on was the awareness of the seductive temptation to explore the provocative behavior that challenged the frame. He wanted me to criticize him. I felt quietly but deeply bad for this damaged young man. I knew that I wanted to rescue him from his privileged prison.

He gradually, in stages over several years, revealed the nature of his relationship with his mother and father, which caused him enormous shame, rage and ill-defined anguish. Each time, I was taken aback by the stories and wondered at times whether he was making them up, being melodramatic—as his mother had suggested he was when she interviewed me—but I came to trust the truthfulness of the meaning of his experience to him.

His mother has been a volatile, fragile, depressed, and raging alcoholic for most of his life. She would scream, hit, control, prohibit his activities that did not fit with her picture of the family. She controlled his contact with his father, and also, in his early adolescence in the years after the divorce, she was sexually provocative and without appropriate boundaries. These occurred at times when she was both sober and drunk. She would punish him for failing to comply with her edicts and then lavish him with expensive clothes, trips, etc. He grew up terrified of her, and only in adolescence became aware of her rage for which he was the only target. He threatened as a teenager to kill himself if she did not stop yelling at him. But he never acted on any of these feelings.

Even as he gradually moved out and on, she would call, demanding submission and compliance with family events, meetings with her to discuss money and obligations. He remained overtly compliant, terrorized and secretly defiant in a pathetically immature and basically masochistic manner. He would get drunk or stoned, go to strip clubs, spend days at video games and not venture out of what he considered the golden prison of his family life.

During these early years, I recognized the temptation to be punitive, strict with him; many times, as I waited for him, I considered saying something like: "You need to sit up so we can talk about what is going on with your missing sessions, lateness, etc. Do you want this analysis or not?" And I would have a chilling sense of unwittingly living out a scene in his head and saying to myself: "Oh great!"

As our relationship deepened, he allowed himself to feel and acknowledge that he was more attached to me. He spoke of it as "the portable doctor G." Interestingly, we discovered and developed a vernacular, as all analyses do, and ours was "the movies"—we both love them and they became ways for us to connect, communicate, diffuse, amuse and detoxify pain at times. He described the experience of his mother's calls as like the scene in the original *Manchurian Candidate* when the mother, played by Angela Lansbury, calls her son, played by Laurence Harvey, and says "Why don't you play a game of solitaire?" Sometimes we were characters in *The Godfather* or *Star Wars*, often with an amusing but painful heroic quality. I was to offer him useful forms of wisdom in his efforts to face the challenges of adult life.

Interlaced with the emergence of the abuse pattern and the cinematic myths were attempts by him to move forward into "his own life." Decisions were very difficult. Whatever he might choose confronted him with the dilemma that nothing would ever be enough to undo his inadequacy or validate his specialness. Anything in what he came to accept as the real world outside the family universe had limitations. Woven into this was the problem of time; the clock ticked and life moved on. Nothing he could do would be great enough to repair, validate or glorify his damaged self-image. Money, prizes, etc., all required facing the world the next day. So why bother trying. You might imagine the countertransference wishes to rescue him from this dilemma, to get him out into the world, doing anything that might allow him to test himself and feel his own agency and autonomy. I felt painful frustration about "if only he would try, if only he would sustain the effort," if only I could free him enough for him to succeed in taking responsibility for himself in the "real world." I hoped to free him from his golden prison. In all of this, I remained painfully and cautiously aware of the depth of his self-identification with both of his self-indulgent parents. Too much therapeutic zeal would serve to deny the intensity of these unconscious identifications.

I had all sorts of countertransference experiences in the course of this treatment: anger, frustration, envy of his financial freedom, pleasure in his misery, outrage at the abuse he suffered, a wish to protect him, to make him strong, even to have him reward me with a named professorship at the institute from the family money.

A particularly telling meaning of this man's masochistic/narcissistic perverse attachment to a traumatic unconscious relationship revealed itself after an especially meaningful experience with his fiancée in which they felt deeply close to each other. She felt grief and mourning for her long-dead mother who would not be at their wedding. Unconsciously, his experience of her attachment to her dead, idealized mother prompted him to feel persecuted and a need to "be on his own." He had a flood of feeling of wanting to be on his own and punish all the women in his life. He recognized that he was just beginning to actually feel "on his own," that is, in charge of his own life and decisions. He saw the intensity of his infantile rage, vindictiveness and ultimate sadness. He felt strange relief. He recognized that he had avoided being able to love someone, needing to feel like a brooding superhero, overcoming his adversaries.

Some weeks after these sessions, he arrived late and was furious because he had actually tried to get to the session on time. In a moment that surprised us both, because lateness was a chronic issue, he started to cry (not usual for him) and described how sad he felt that he had treated himself and me in this "shabby fashion." With deepening poignancy and grief, he told me how grateful he truly was for the treatment and to me. Just as he was afraid of loving and losing his fiancée, he knew that he had been afraid to acknowledge how much he loved me. We were both deeply moved. It was a moment in which I felt tearful and knew there was nothing I needed to say.

They married, moved away, had children, and, as I learned from letters over the years, they learned to deal with life without extra pain and suffering.

CONCLUSION

Rethinking our understanding of masochistic character structure offers a valuable opportunity to examine both our psychoanalytic models of mental life and of therapeutic action. The notion of the pursuit of misery, and of motivated suffering, demands an appreciation of the tenacious power of primitive unconscious fantasy. This is most evident in the impact of early traumatic object relations on ego structure and self-organization and regulation.

The analysis of unconscious guilt most always plays a significant therapeutic role in masochistic clinical phenomena. However, when early trauma and or severe narcissistic pathology are aspects of the clinical presentation or emerge in the course of treatment, I have found it extremely helpful to remember the primitivity of the superego function and the profundity of primitive unconscious attachments. Guilt serves deeper purposes in the maintenance of such fragile identifications and self-regulation. Nowhere is this more crucial than in problematic transference-countertransference reactions that come to dominate the analytic and therapeutic process.

I have found the following clinical observations essential in my work with masochistic character phenomena:

Constant attention to the question—why does the patient want to hold on to this pain or impoverishment, this empty life rather than have success or pleasure? What makes this better? What does it preserve and protect? What ideal self is maintained this way? What victory is maintained, what guilt or destruction is avoided?

The profound role of secrets. The analyst is the last to know! Perhaps more than most neurotic structures, the masochist has the biggest investment in secret-keeping; once the patient has engaged and established the needed masochistic (sadomasochistic) transference, any shift, any little success, pleasure, assertion, non-victimized experience must be kept secret from the analyst! If you demand to know, if you pressure the patient to reveal their secret satisfactions, they will victoriously destroy them and reveal you to be the narcissistic demanding, selfish object they always assumed you were! Gains from the treatment are fragile; they can feel like they are written in sand or made of smoke. This is the essence of the "negative therapeutic reaction."

In the most general sense, the treatment works to the extent that it can work through the very slow, patient submission to the patient's need to preserve their masochism, through the tolerance, persistence, lack of traumatizing imposition of the analyst's perceived demands (like getting better), the long slow disconfirmation of the transference, the incremental internalization of robust, benign, independent super-ego representation, a new object relationship, and/ or new self-self-object. What comes through over the long haul is the impact of the relationship, the analyst as steward of some modified sense of self that is not wedded to or defined by suffering and unhappiness and the virtue of pain. That's the simple story of how this works!

It requires "infinite" patience, humility, unrelenting curiosity and unfailing respect for the patient's internal world and psychic reality as well as eternal vigilance for the demoralizing effect on the analyst, feelings of deadness, hopelessness and powerlessness and the inevitable counter-transference reactions that arise from a denial of our sadism, the wish to rescue or be rescued or the more naked expression of our sadism = our wish to punish, beat, humiliate, subjugate, or cruelly abandon the patient and thereby live out our identifications with the patient's wished-for projections.

NOTE

1. See Glick and Meyers (1988), chapter 1 for a further elaboration of Freud's theories of masochism and the subsequent history of psychoanalytic theories of masochism.

REFERENCES

Cooper, A. M. (1988). The narcissistic masochistic character. In *Masochism: Current Clinical Perspectives,* eds. R. A. Glick and D. I. Meyers. Hillsdale, NJ: Analytic Press, 117–38.

Freud, S. (1905). Three essays on sexuality. *Standard Edition* 7: 135–243.

——— (1924). The economic problem of masochism. *Standard Edition* 19: 159–70.

Glick, R. A., and Meyers, D. I. (1988). *Masochism: Current Clinical Perspectives.* Hillsdale, NJ: Analytic Press.

Krafft-von Ebing, R. von (1906). *Psychopathia Sexuali.* New York Physicians & Surgeons Books Co., 1931

Sacher-Masoch, L. R. von (1870). *Venus in Furs.* New York: W. Faro, 1932.

Schafer, R. (1988). Those wrecked by success. In *Masochism: Current Clinical Perspectives,* eds. R. A. Glick and D. I. Meyers. Hillsdale, NJ: Analytic Press, 81–91.

FIVE

Sadomasochistic Stuckness

Stanley J. Coen, MD

A highly skilled psychoanalyst told me about a session with a patient who feared she would get into sadomasochistic struggle with her mother. My colleague described her efforts to divert her patient from struggling with her mother by play-acting with the patient, using various tactics to keep the mother from exploding at her. This was unusual treatment behavior for my colleague. I sensed her discomfort with her patient's wish to struggle with her mother provocatively because it stirred similar vulnerability and temptation in my colleague. I tried to help her with this while I was well aware that this situation seemed too threatening for her. This is a simple example from a very good analyst. Hence I think this example is relevant to many of us. In these typical situations, analyst and patient would probably not be able to explore productively the patient's fascination with sadomasochistic struggle.

A fine supervisee beginning a new analysis felt concerned about how angry she had been feeling at her patient's controlling struggle with her about getting a consultation with a psychopharmacologist. She acknowledged that she has needed to work on her anger at her patient in her own analysis. Partly, she felt she should just insist that her new patient follow her recommendation to consult with a psychopharmacologist, just listen to her and stop fighting with her. She believed she should not be feeling so angry with her patient, and that her anger had to be neurotic. She felt critical of his narcissistic entitlement, demandingness and selfishness. She felt like pathologizing him. Indeed, she felt like a controlling mother. From the process material she presented, it became clear to me that indeed this was the opening up of her patient's transference; he engaged her intensely, and angrily, as if she really were the controlling mother. Of course, she was also the "good" mother, but she had to tolerate switching rapidly between both roles without too much discomfort. Her patient needed to be able to fight with her, hate her, criticize her, and draw her in closely through such struggle. No longer was the immediate issue whether to demand that he get the psychopharmacological consultation or to drop the issue but for her to stay with the intense struggle between them. This was the sudden deepening of this treatment. But she had to be able to tolerate being hated and hating her new patient as well as being pulled at by him so as to intensify their bond.

It has been painful to hear many capable analysts and therapists display their shame at having been drawn into sadomasochistic interactions with patients rather than to take for granted, with more equanimity, that they will have to experience this with some patients. When the analyst can feel his own temptations to be drawn into sadomasochistic struggle with patients, then he is much better prepared to talk with them about what they are bringing into the treatment room. The more analysts can feel their own sadomasochistic temptations, the more they can head off gross enactments with patients—at least to a degree. When analysts are too anxious about their and their patients' hostile aggression, it can be very tempting to manage their anxiety via sadomasochistic struggle. Sadomasochism is much safer than outright hatred and destructiveness, since it is covered over by seductive, sexual, or even some loving feelings. Patients and analysts may feel anxious about their temptations to be drawn into sadomasochistic struggle.

Most patients and therapists find it difficult to actually feel (not think) their own wishes to be involved in or remain in destructive and self-destructive battle with another person. It is easy to understand that other people might want to fight with their spouse or parents so as to feel intensely connected to them. But it can be very difficult to actually allow oneself to feel a wish to struggle with another person so as not to be autonomous and responsible for oneself. That feeling is what makes it so difficult for pathologically dependent sadomasochistic patients to change. Analysts may want to believe that they have analyzed their sadomasochistic temptations in their training analysis or reanalysis, and therapists may believe that they have mastered their sadomasochistic temptations in their own treatments, and that they have somehow magically purged this out of themselves. The Novicks (1987) emphasized the difficulty in masochism of relinquishing the preoedipal tie to the mother. To the degree that one is afraid of being separate, it remains very tempting to demonstrate one's disability to another person, who is to stand in for the parent. Then the patient remains tempted to display what is wrong, to fail, to be inept, so as to invite the other one as parent to take over. That is what I want the reader to see in the patient I'll tell about in detail. Such patients may emphasize their anxiety and insecurity, which are real, while remaining out of touch with their eager willingness not to become capable in their own right. I emphasize patients' stuckness so as to be able to focus analyst and patient on what stuck patients need to contend with. Otherwise, like the patient I describe, they can just persist in staying in the same place, unable to focus on what is wrong. What is wrong remains external so that it is someone else's job—the analyst's—to fix it.

In the case vignette that follows, I encourage the reader to identify with my struggles, in order to help prepare for those aspects of sadomasochistic engagement to which you may be most vulnerable. I fully believe that identifying with an "analyst-in-trouble" (Coen, 2010b) can be very helpful for clinicians so as to catch their own temptations and vulnerabilities. To do so, you will need to fight against the self-protective urge to insist that my difficulties could not have been your own.

I could feel impatient that after these many years, and many treatments, Ms. B. initiate, remember, make some connection to previous sessions, to problems within herself—or more unreasonably on my part— show some willingness to explore herself, take some responsibility for her conflicts. Songs frequently went through Ms. B.'s mind, but she feared letting me in on them and often would not do so. Remember the old song, "Enjoy yourself, it's later than you think?" In Ms. B.'s presence, I would often think "Explore yourself, it's later than you think!" I could get caught up in struggle with Ms. B. about how her treatment needed to proceed, making it difficult for me to grasp that she had needed to learn to insist, to fight about her needs being met. It was easy to justify this as her refusal to do the work of the treatment, which indeed she would not do. Ms. B.'s multiple other therapists had threatened to end her treatment because of her lack of focus on what she herself wanted to work out. She would arrive for her sessions at the last minute, bring all of her things into the consulting room and then remove her outer garments and her shoes which she would drop by the chair. It was a kind of nonsexual striptease—or at least nothing sexual was to be attributed to it. She would fold her feet under her on the chair or stretch her legs across the arm of the chair as if she were a young child who was curling up. When I replaced the old recliner chair with a somewhat smaller stationary leather chair, she was furious that I'd gotten rid of her comfortable chair without consulting her. She insisted I should have taken her along with me in selecting the new chair. It took some time before she could acknowledge the repetition in her transference feelings of her mother not consulting her in redecorating her room while she was away at camp.

She would complain about what was wrong in her life, wanting practical advice on how to deal with life's exigencies, which she contended I would never provide for her. Ms. B. refused to deal with her imaginings, fantasies, dreams, which she insisted was all I was interested in, not in her. She was irritable, critical, dissatisfied, dark, edgy. For most of our many years of work together, Ms. B. fought against allowing intense needs, longings or desires, which made her feel vulnerable, into the room between us. Sexual feelings were especially frightening. Just before coming to me, she fired a colleague after the initial consultation for ogling her breasts. He became "the molester." I was not to look at and enjoy her body or talk about sex or her defenses against it. When I would walk into the room after her, she'd hiss that I was looking at her ass. She'd protest if I tried to open up our exploring how this would work. She did not want to have any of those "creepy" wishes, which sometimes she did have with me.

She had good reason to feel bitter, pessimistic, and mistrustful of relations with others. She grew up with rejection, neglect, deprivation and battles with each parent about whose needs were to be satisfied. Our struggles about working at the treatment, remembering sessions, making connections, exploring fantasies and analyzing dreams repeated in the transference struggles with her mother. She could feel like her father's beautiful princess until her developing sexuality collided with his phallic narcissism; he talked too much about her developing body and his own sexuality.

When I could not keep in mind how terrified she was to change, get better, become more capable of functioning on her own, I would resent rather than empathize with her refusal. At such times, I too was refusing to resonate with what persists of regressive temptations in myself. Her willingness to remain stuck and feel disabled, needed to be engaged patiently, slowly. I also felt stuck, unable to grasp what we were doing with each other. The more responsible I could become for my own temptations to regress, to join in battle with her, to connect intensely but negatively, the more easily could I step outside of them. Then I could resonate with our temptations to struggle with each other, while not giving in to them, so that I could help her much more effectively to do so, too.

Psychoanalysts—all therapists—do not readily acknowledge their own wishes to regress. When I (Coen, 2000) presented an earlier paper on the topic, one discussant insisted he never had such wishes. Only one colleague confided to me that he too had experienced similar regressive temptations. But I also was surprised to discover my regressive temptations, evoked in resonance with my patient's. Rosemary Balsam (1997), a discussant of an earlier paper of mine (Coen, 1997), was able to show me, in a way that I could accept, that I had joined my patient in mutual regression to a pathological maternal object. I mean by this that both my patient and I felt helpless and defeated, as if neither of us could care for ourselves or for the other without active provision from a mother. I had temporarily joined my patient in a form of regressive relatedness that promises relief from conflict. In doing so I *temporarily* ceded my role as constructive therapist who contains and interprets. The psychopharmacologist helped both of us, to a degree, out of our negativism. I found it difficult to tolerate my helplessness to interpret effectively to my patient while he was in his regression. Of course, I knew that when a patient becomes very regressed, the therapist has to tolerate, contain and sustain the treatment until the patient can again become a therapeutic collaborator. But I was too willing to give up, for which I hated my patient and myself, and to join my patient in wanting someone (a mother) to rescue us. I had consciously expected to experience regressive temptations only with psychotic patients. This is very different from my current position. I now expect that, in order to help free up my stuck masochistic patients, I need to resample my own wishes to feel disabled. Once I can connect with this again, then I can empathically and confidently talk with my patients about their wishes to remain hobbled.

Our work together was made easier by Ms. B.'s ambivalence, by the fact that her positive, caring feelings came across, despite her intense negativism, more clearly than from any of my other intensely negativistic patients. Early in her treatment, I had to be out for a couple of weeks over Christmas/New Years for a minor surgical procedure. She was my only patient who sent flowers with a warm note. Given her negativism and anxiety about caring, I was touched and surprised that she was able to do so.

Here is an example from early in the treatment of Ms. B. and I working well together at analyzing her sadomasochism. She began her session terrified that she was going crazy and needed to be hospitalized. Feeling unable to manage her work and her life, she proceeded to give me examples of how poorly she was functioning. Feeling panicky, depressed and hopeless, she insisted she could not cope with the exigencies of life. She needed a hospital. By the end of the session, we had moved to Ms. B.'s being able to own her wishes to go crazy, regress and have me care for her full-time. By then, she had became able to tolerate and enjoy her dramatic performance in her regressive crisis. The more she got into her rage-filled demand that I care for her totally, the more she was able to feel and connect her current wishes to regress with her bitter feelings of deprivation, neglect and misuse by her parents. As this session progressed, she and I were able to get hold of her sadomasochistic desires to torment me with her failure and falling apart, to blame me and make me responsible for her and for her difficulties. I was able to use my own feelings of being blamed, tortured and attacked to engage her about her pleasure in what she was doing with me. We were able to turn the nightmare scenario with which she began into a kind of theater that we could both enjoy and discuss, as we became the audience rather than the actors. The more crazy and suicidal she became, the more she would cause her parents and me to suffer. She talked about giving up her job and managing on her savings. The last four days she hadn't bothered to shower. Should she let herself regress further and insist that I fully take over her care? She mused that some believe it's therapeutic for patients to regress as fully as possible.

Now she felt much better, as she owned her wishes to regress further in order to torture her parents and me. She was no longer terrified of going crazy and requiring hospitalization. She wanted me to accept her just as she was without any interpretation of defense, so she would not have to experience me as a dissatisfied, critical parent who relentlessly insisted she do more in the treatment. She enjoyed feeling dependent on me, wanting me to care for her and love her so much more. Ms. B. ended the session pleased with how much she had been able to let herself go in indulging her wishes to regress, attack and torture me. This contrasted with her panicky conviction earlier in the session that she was *actually* going crazy. Ms. B.'s wish to go crazy and be hospitalized made her feel less anxiously responsible for her desires that I care for her. That she needed to be cared for because of her childhood deprivation felt much safer than her wanting me to care for and love her, which made her feel "creepy" in my presence. She feared feeling intense desire toward me, afraid that I would misuse her sexually.

But I could once again be surprised and unaccepting of those times when she again became unreasonable in sessions, when she didn't want to be at her session, talk, think, do anything. I could immediately feel angry that she didn't make any connection with where she had just been emotionally or with what had just been going on in her treatment. I could think to myself that she should, at least intellectually, be able to make some connection. Sometimes, I missed her anger at me expressed through such refusal. Then we struggled with each other. Of course, intellectually I could grasp that when she was very angry with me or afraid of progress and close loving feelings, she would defend herself by becoming unreasonable and negativistic.

But she didn't only express anger at me by being unreasonable. She also wanted to struggle with me sadomasochistically. She would spit out the word, "pressure," sometimes when I'd made an interpretation, sometimes even when I'd been quiet and patient. At first, I felt that I needed to be very tolerant of her sensitivity to being impinged upon by the angry, critical, needy mother or the phallic, narcissistic father. If she sensed that I needed something from her, she'd feel angry and threatened. It was very difficult to explore sexual feelings because she became very anxious, emphasizing her fear of my impinging on her. She was aware how anxious it made her to feel sexually aroused, but she was very hesitant to explore in herself why that was so. It became clear that her hissing the word "pressure" was also an invitation for us to fight, putting me in the role of the bad, impinging parent. Of course, she'd had much reason to resent this aspect of her parents. But she also wanted to connect with me and her partner through what was wrong, and struggle about it. Sometimes, her excitement in such sadomasochistic struggle began to feel sexual to her. It became clear that when she felt signs of change, progress, and close, loving feelings, she became anxious. Then she would return to sadomasochistic struggle, which felt like a much safer way to stay connected.

Even though we worked together for a long time and separation was such a major issue for her, each time she would begin to feel disrupted by a separation, she would insist that was not happening, that this was my theme. She would struggle for quite some time as each separation approached that this was not what was bothering her. I'd have to remind her that this was how she dealt with separation each time it occurred, while she would continue to deny it. Eventually, she would get very caught up in intense feelings about being left on her own; then she would be amazed that she hadn't let herself grasp this. What seemed to help most was my attitude, which I sometimes interpreted and sometimes contained, that in her refusal to participate with me, she was demonstrating how angry she felt at my leaving her, like when her parents would go away when she was little. I could not return and just expect her to be reasonable with me as her parents seem to have insisted. When I welcomed her resentment toward me as essential, as expressed by her refusal, she would feel better, feel more acceptable in her anger. When I, like her parents, wanted her to behave more reasonably, she became much more antagonistic.

I had to keep moving between different attitudes towards her. Here I needed to be accepting of her unreasonableness and her refusal as legitimately expressing her resentment at separation between us. She was an angry woman who had much difficulty acknowledging her anger. She would insist that she was not angry, that she didn't see herself as angry, that I was making this up. But she used denial very broadly, so that she tended to repudiate most of her difficulties.

Fairly early in the treatment she was able to work her way out of her feelings that she couldn't succeed at her career. Although she was now freer to enjoy her work, which became a relatively safe island, she continued to feel disabled otherwise. She continued to insist on her own ineptness, for which others should and would criticize and reject her. We could now talk about her willingness to play the role of the disappointing child who would get attention through her apparent disability and her fears of competing with her siblings, parents and me. She insisted on her disability as a woman and as a patient. Invariably another—a sister or a good friend—would be the attractive, appealing woman who would take men away from her. She'd insist on what was wrong with her body. She focused on how awful and unattractive her body was with the sense that she needed to be punished. It was difficult for her to imagine herself as the woman who could win the man. She was afraid to picture herself as my protégé, my favorite; she couldn't be an appealing patient; her siblings were much better patients. Given what we knew of her siblings' problems, in and out of treatment, this perception was a break with reality. She could easily spoil the good feelings between us by insisting that

I was going to interpret too deeply, too sexually. She was afraid to allow herself to enjoy good feelings with her partner and with me. It was very hard for her to be satisfied. She was much more comfortable focusing on what was wrong than on what was right.

Sometimes it was difficult to know whether she was into sadomasochistic fighting or we were reliving feelings that her legitimate needs had been insufficiently acknowledged by either parent, and sometimes we would shift quickly from one to the other. Indeed, she remained furious at her emotional neglect as a child by both parents which she expressed with me. The provocative way in which she did this made it seem that she wanted to fight with me rather than "more legitimately" express her chronic rage. She tended to be surprised at her angry refusal to collaborate with me when she and I had been doing well together. She wanted her angry feelings to go away. Sometimes I could want that too. Then we had trouble.

Given how vulnerable Ms. B. was to feeling intruded upon, used for the other person's needs, I had to be highly sensitive to not imposing my ways on her. We worked best when I was able to keep what was transpiring between us implicit rather than interpret it too closely. When I told her a week before that we would not meet Memorial Day, she hit the roof. She was enraged that I was taking time off, then leaving her on vacation. Why wouldn't I work Memorial Day, some Saturdays, and Sundays to make this up to her? Eventually she calmed down and told me of good experiences from the previous Saturday, including a passing reference to feeling good thinking of me. She then became anxious and avoidant, only later revealing she had thought that I was the best man she had ever met. She sobbed, afraid she would now feel too vulnerable.

Two days after Memorial Day, she arrived enraged, desperate, anxious: "Without you, I'd leave my partner!" She began complaining about him at length. I told her she was safer focusing on what she was not getting from him than from me. She calmed down when I told her she had blocked out missing and feeling enraged with me. Despite the uproar she caused in the session, I was effective in telling her that she was avoiding and displacing her rage at me for not having been available for her. She seemed angrily excited as she described going after the person who had been unavailable and unresponsive so as to be able to draw that person—me—in. The next day she wore a bright orange top, more revealing than usual. I was struck by the color in contrast to her persistent black; she was in a good mood. I liked her like this. She appreciated how I helped her yesterday. She dreamed she was with a woman friend. She thought of R. who rejected her as a teen, then of J. who was in a postpartum depression. The woman and she were very close in the dream, hugging; the woman seemed to kiss her on the teeth. The closeness felt good, like merging. The woman only spent a little time with her, had others to be with. She said nothing about the dream directly. It felt too close to have a session today after yesterday. I said she didn't seem uncomfortable with feeling close in the dream. The mood in the session changed. She became silent; I now felt her to be remote and rejecting. Had allowing herself to appreciate my help and wanting to come closer to me led her to fear that I would then disappoint her so that she needed to retreat? I no longer felt effective with her. I said that the woman in the dream in a post-partum depression couldn't respond well to her child. She told about her mother not helping her when other girls taunted her; she painted a picture of an unhelpful mother. I said we both seemed to think that yesterday I wasn't an unhelpful mother at all but that I seemed to have become one. She ignored my encouragement to wonder about what had happened between us.

She dreamed, immediately after another break, about being with her brother and a much younger blond girl. Her brother and the girl were flirting. The girl kissed her brother. Ms. B. yelled at her to stop doing that. Her brother, accepting of what the girl was doing, didn't stop it. She didn't associate to her dream. I thought we needed not to pin this down too much. I said it was good that she was opening herself up, allowing herself to feel longings. She objected: she doesn't let herself feel longings; they're dangerous, scary. Wearing a body suit in the session, her thighs were fully exposed. She reported that she had flirted with a seventy-year-old dentist, enjoying his attention, but that he was old enough to be her father or grandfather. She thought I called the seventy-year-old dentist a seventy-year-old analyst; I seemed to be saying that I was feeling sexually attracted to her. I said that she had been adamant there were to be no sexual feelings in this treatment room; she was now a bit more comfortable with wanting to be my favorite patient, but it was still scary.

I tried to use a light touch toward the emotional resonance in the air between us without fully interpreting it in words. By my not interpreting her longings too much in relation to me, they came into the room. It was as if I were to be the accepting father (and mother) who enjoyed her as a sexually developing girl, his princess, without throwing sexuality, hers and his, in her face. I was to see what she revealed and enjoy it without calling too much attention to it. For example, she dreamed: "I keep taking off my shirt as I want to get attention from a man. My body feels and looks good to me." She did not associate to her dream nor did I try to interpret it, only to acknowledge that she was taking a chance in allowing us to see good in her.

COMMENTARY ON MY CASE

I have emphasized how my own regressive, sadomasochistic temptations could get in my way in working with Ms. B. I have done so deliberately so as to enable the reader to identify with me as an "analyst-in-trouble" in order to catch your own similar temptations. Of course, I was also the capable, effective analyst who enjoyed and helped his patient. If patient and analyst need to live out their conflicts with each other, then they cannot analyze them. To the degree that the therapist can catch and contain his interfering conflicts, he can then assist his patient to do so, too. To the degree that clinicians are ashamed and intolerant of their persistent regressive, sadomasochistic wishes, they may blame the patient for what is wrong in the treatment—the presence of intense regressive, sadomasochism within the affective force-field between them.

Once the clinician can catch, tolerate and contain his own contribution to what is wrong within the treatment, he can then more empathically focus on and talk with his patient about her difficulties. But with a patient like Ms. B., who is so afraid to change, grow, and become autonomous and self-sufficient, much of the analytic work has to be about stuckness, clinging, refusal, disability. If the clinician cannot tolerate his own similar regressive wishes to fail, be inept, dependent, defeated, he won't be able to tolerate his patient's intense need not to use analysis productively. When I felt under pressure to get my patient not to be herself, not to be an "anti-analysand," I would stir her up even further. It was so easy to rationalize this, as her previous therapists had also done, as necessary for the success of the treatment. Then, of course, she objected vigorously that I cared about "the treatment" rather than about her. On the other hand, when I could talk with her empathically—for her not for me—then we could talk usefully about her wish to remain stuck forever.

My patient needed to struggle with me. Exciting sadomasochistic struggle brought her connection to the other, which she craved, and protection against separation, loneliness, and hatred, which she dreaded. In such struggle, she did not have to own responsibly how much she craved close connection with others. Threats of separation especially stirred up sadomasochistic struggle. When she acknowledged her intense, needy cravings for others, she felt very vulnerable, panicky. To make herself feel safer, she would then deny her neediness. Feeling appreciative and loving led her to feel terrified of how much she now cared about the other person, who could reject or respond to her. Either prospect was terrifying. She would regularly regress from a loving stance back to a more sadomasochistic one. Exciting struggle tempted her as being far better than feeling depressed, lonely and neglected. She longed to engage others to provide her with what they, and everyone else before, had failed to give her. Deprived and mistreated, she felt entitled to have her needs met. Ms. B. refused to acknowledge that she could want too much from others, that it was not true that friends cheated her by talking about themselves some of the time. The problem, as she saw it, was that the world failed to provide for her needs which she had to remedy. Despite this attitude, she had felt depressed for most of her life, experiencing herself as insufficient and inadequate.

Even when her dreams, associations, her narration in the session and what she wanted from me pointed clearly to how much she craved a mother to care for her, she would get angry at such interpretation. This sort of intervention was very different from acknowledging with her how neglected she had felt by her mother and how misused she had felt by her father. That she had good reason to feel angry made her feel supported, even if she then had to deny that she was an angry person. She wanted me and others to provide for her without her having to acknowledge her intense neediness.

I still believe (Coen, 1988) that the temptation of exciting struggle with the other person makes sadomasochism very difficult to relinquish. I wrote (Coen, 1992, p. 193): "It is exciting to feel able to induce intense affective responses in another person, to overcome the other's barriers, to feel in control and dominant, able to make the other feel bad, guilty, weak, inferior, defective. It is exciting to hold another person in the palm of one's hand, to push another to the point of losing control, attacking, leaving, and then to be reassured that this will not occur." I would now also emphasize how provocative struggle with the other person achieves connection without the vulnerability inherent in acknowledging need for the other. Neediness can appear in a negative form, in which the manifest aim seems to be avoidance of all need. Such patients obscure their dependency by camouflaging it behind negative, provocative, angry engagement with others. I (Coen, 2010a) have called this "negative neediness" because it disavows the patient's neediness while drawing in the other person through struggle about what is wrong. Patient and therapist, if similarly susceptible in their struggles, may hide from themselves and miss the intensity of their need for close connection with each other. It is not news that this is an aspect of sadomasochism, but clinicians need to be prepared to recognize that it may be much safer for patient and therapist to connect negatively rather than more lovingly (also see Coen, 1994).

And I still believe that pathological dependency is central to such patients' terror of managing on their own. I wrote (Coen, 1992, p. 194):

> Instead of facing what has been wrong, the patient becomes excited in repeating what a parent (mother) did with one. Indeed, the excited, erotized repetition serves to ward off the horrors of destructiveness, mother's and one's own. Erotization tames destructiveness; one can pretend that it is a kind of loving relatedness, an exciting game sought by both participants. This is very different from acknowledging that one person hates, envies, and begrudges another his own life, his own separateness and autonomy, and wants to destroy this.

I now want to emphasize, more than I have done previously, patients' fear of change in the treatment which they must oppose. Ms. B. could refuse, fight, struggle against what she imagined I wanted from her in the treatment. She was afraid to be my collaborator and to want to get better in her treatment. Any change, especially for the better, threatened her with loss of the status quo and with abandonment in a world in which she feared that she could not manage on her own. I now tolerate patients' unreasonableness and refusal to collaborate much better than I did once upon a time. I am now more prepared to be patient over a very long time with patients who are afraid to change. I have had to find my way between such patient tolerance and empathic ways of helping my patients to engage their stuckness.

Indeed such stuckness is awful. It is awful for patients to so fear autonomy that they will do anything to avoid it, to seek any way of being connected to another, especially when this connection threatens to destroy autonomy and competence. But patients cannot be forced by their therapists to change. Of course, we all know that. But it is easy for the therapist to become pressuring, insistent that the patient be reasonable and address his problems, including his stuckness. That will only make the situation worse. Such patients do need to feel accepted and contained by their psychoanalysts and therapists over a long time before it becomes possible to talk with them about the pathology of their stuckness. And even once the analytic couple is able to address the stuckness, there will be inevitable oscillations backward and forward, periods of struggle as well as of collaboration. The therapist's needs of the patient—to be reasonable, change, improve—will anger the patient. When the therapist is seen as the needy parent, mother or father, the patient has to refuse further.

I (Coen, 1992, chapter 15) have previously presented an impassioned plea for psychoanalysts to engage the stuckness of pathologically dependent patients so as to help them move forward. I emphasized analysts' hesitation and difficulties with rage and destructiveness, just like their patients', which can keep the analytic couple from fully engaging what is wrong in the treatment. Some colleagues objected that analyses, at least analyses done by them, need not be as stormy as I reported. I still believe that analyzing rage, hatred and destructivenss are essential to loosening pathologically dependent bonds. But I now want to shift the analytic burden more toward the therapist's side, even more than I (Coen, 2002) have previously done. I believe that to help free up stuck sadomasochistic, pathologically dependent patients requires that the therapist empathically tolerate feeling similar regressive temptations in himself to those of his patients. It has to be painful for analyzed clinicians to have to tolerate wishes to fail, to be inept, disabled. By feeling their own similar regressive wishes, therapists can then help patients bear, with less critical attack, their patients' wishes to remain stuck, incapable. Otherwise, it is tempting for therapists to disown their regressive temptations, to put them into their patients, and then to self-righteously berate their patients for the stuck treatment.

Psychoanalysts do not easily talk about their temptations with their patients (Jacobson, 2010). Talking about and writing about our universal temptations — with our patients, within ourselves — is aimed at encouraging colleagues to explore and bear what they would otherwise disclaim so as to help our stuck patients to do the same. This is not merely a relational way of connecting with more difficult patients. If therapists cannot go to where the patient needs to go, they cannot succeed. Colleagues, just like their patients, may need reassurance that they can have regressive, sadomasochistic temptations and still function very well as highly competent autonomous adults. Then they can assist their patients to do so, too. It is so freeing, for analyst and patient, to gain the confidence that they can move in and out of regressive, sadomasochistic wishes, without becoming trapped in them forever. The same goes for loving and for hating feelings. Therapist and patient need to be able to feel confidently that they can come as close as they wish lovingly or want to murder hatefully without resultant *action* — boundary crossing or violation, permanent fusion or death. Then feelings and wishes can be reversible, safer, and even enjoyable.

REFERENCES

Balsam, R. (1997 unpublished). Discussion of "How to help patients (and analysts) bear the unbearable." *Association for Psychoanalytic Medicine,* New York.

Coen, S. J. (1988). Sadomasochistic excitement. In *Masochism: Current Psychoanalytic Views,* eds. R. A. Glick and D. I. Meyers. Hillsdale, NJ: Analytic Press, 43–59.

——— (1992). *The Misuse of Persons: Analyzing Pathological Dependency.* Hillsdale, NJ and London: Analytic Press.

——— (1994). Barriers to love between patient and analyst. *Journal of the American Psychoanalytic Association* 42: 1107–35.

——— (1997). How to help patients (and analysts) bear the unbearable. *Journal of the American Psychoanalytic Association* 45: 1183–207.

——— (2000). The wish to regress in patient and analyst. *Journal of the American Psychoanalytic Association* 48: 785–810.

——— (2002). *Affect Intolerance in Patient and Analyst.* Northvale, NJ: Jason Aronson.

——— (2010a). Neediness and narcissistic defensive action. *Psychoanalytic Quarterly* 79: 969–90.

——— (2010b) Book review essay: Rereading Masud Khan today: Have his writings fallen with him? *Journal of the American Psychoanalytic Association* 58: 1005–20.

Jacobson, W. (2010). Behind the couch: Uses and misuses of temptation. *Journal of the American Psychoanalytic Association* 58: 1189–99.

Novick, K. K., and Novick, J. (1987). The essence of masochism. *Psychoanalytic Study of the Child* 42: 53–84.

SIX

Masochism as a
Multiply-Determined Phenomenon

Glen O. Gabbard, MD

Over twenty years ago, I heard Otto Kernberg speak to a group of analysts on the subject of masochism. The paper was scholarly and comprehensive. I remember thinking that the scope of his impressive overview made it seem as though most forms of human behavior fell under the rubric of masochistic activity. I was a bit skeptical at the time, but after nearly thirty-five years of clinical experience, I find myself in substantial agreement with Kernberg's notion that masochistic phenomena are pervasive, a position that was also expressed over thirty years ago in a panel on masochism at the American Psychoanalytic Association meeting. I am frankly amazed by the human propensity to unconsciously seek out tormenting experiences. I am also increasingly aware of the multiple and complex determinants of masochistic desires and behavior. Masochistic phenomena rarely can be reduced to one unconscious conflict or one developmental moment. Analysts must be prepared to find a confluence of factors that converge in the masochistic symptoms and to discover that much of the self-defeating behavior is surprisingly ego-syntonic.

We have moved beyond the idea that masochism should be narrowly construed as only a perversion in which one gains pleasure from pain. For most masochistically organized individuals, it is more useful clinically to see them as having a need to experience painful, humiliating and self-destructive relationships or self-states. Irwin Rosen (1993) wrote of relational masochism, which is fundamentally the search for a "bad enough object." It is not simply that these individuals obtain pleasure from pain. Rather, by seeking out and attaching to objects that will treat them badly, they retain a sense of self-continuity, of intrapsychic organization, even of security and safety. One of the great travesties in the history of official psychiatric nosology is the exclusion of masochistic or self-defeating personality, from the official nomenclature because of political concerns that the suffering of women due to economic and social factors would be regarded as a psychiatric syndrome from which one could infer that women themselves were drawn to suffering. Sacher-Masoch was a poet of male masochism, and in my clinical experience, investment in suffering is just as common, if not more common, in men as it is in women.

Like all behaviors and symptoms, masochistic tendencies are multiply determined. One determinant may relate to active mastery over passively experienced trauma. Patients who re-create the abusive and humiliating experiences from childhood are re-working a traumatic experience, but this time on their own terms with themselves in the driver's seat. Patients with childhood trauma often live with the certainty that lightning will strike again (Bromberg, 1996). Hence they are convinced that feelings of optimism or well-being are dangerously tempting fate. By unconsciously orchestrating the repetition of childhood trauma, they avoid being ambushed by it. Moreover, attaching to an abusive or sadistic object may be better than having no relationship at all.

A common theme in masochism that has guided me through many puzzling clinical situations is this: the masochistic solution is better than something else. Collaborating with the patient in a search for what that "something else" is can be highly productive in disentangling the web of conflicts, defenses, anxieties and problematic internal object relations. Various forms of suffering often defend against anxieties regarding retaliation from oedipal rivals or from primitively based envious attacks (Gabbard, 2000). Fenichel (1945) noted that some of these patients are making a sacrifice—accepting a lesser evil in lieu of castration. The oft-heard exhortation, "break a leg," offered to a performer before going onstage is one such example of making a sacrifice to the gods in hopes of appeasing them and avoiding a worse fate. Helplessness, humiliation and self-pity may also be a cry for help (Cooper, 1993).

I have found Arnold Cooper's work on narcissistic-masochistic personality to be important in how I think about patients with these propensities. Narcissism and masochism are inextricably bound together in so many patients—exemplified by a powerful unconscious fantasy that may be summarized as: "Because of the extraordinary nature of my suffering, I am entitled to special recognition and to exceptions to the rules." Many clinicians who engage in sexual misconduct fit this model (Gabbard and Lester, 2003). They may be well- known in their communities for treating patients who are highly challenging, and they pride themselves on their capacity to "hang in there" with patients who are relentlessly contemptuous and demanding. Sexual contact with patients may result in part from a masochistic surrender to the sadism of the patient with the omnipotent fantasy that by submitting they will "cure" the patient with their self-sacrifice. One forty-four-year-old male therapist who had systematically submitted to the demands of a twenty-eight-year-old borderline patient to prevent her from killing herself ended up having intercourse with her on one occasion. He then reported himself to the ethics committee of his local professional organization. He was surprised at the disciplinary response he received. When he finally consulted me, he looked me in the eye and said: "Everyone focuses on the negative aspects of what I did. Doesn't anyone realize that I saved her from suicide?" In the course of treatment he revealed a lifelong identification with Christ and told me: "It was almost as though I was trying to sacrifice myself so she could live."

The Christ identification underscores the role of grandiosity in masochistic patients. Steven Cooper (no relation to Arnold) has linked self-criticism to unconscious grandiosity as well (2010). He describes patients who engage in excessive self-reproach during the course of the analysis. They may make comments like "I hate myself" or "I'm such a loser" as a form of pre-emptive strike. Because of oedipally based anxieties that father or mother will retaliate against them for their success, they anticipate shaming or humiliating when they do something well. Cooper notes, "Self-criticism may serve as a way to be active rather than passively awaiting an unconsciously shaming experience with an internalized object relation" (2010, pp. 1115–16). Hence some masochistic patients may be saying to the analyst: "Please don't attack me because you can see that I'm already tormenting myself."

In my previous work (Gabbard, 1996, 2000) I have acknowledged my debt to Kleinian thinking in my understanding of masochism. Envy may decimate one's capacity to accept offers of love and help from others (Klein, 1957). Hence such patients often feel shamed and humiliated by the prospect of positive relationships because it makes them acutely aware of those things lacking in themselves that others have. As Bion (1959) put it: "The patient feels he is being allowed an opportunity at which he had hitherto been cheated; the poignancy of his deprivation is thereby rendered the more acute and so are the feelings of resentment at the deprivation." Such individuals must spoil their envy. Masochism and sadism, of course, are two sides of the same coin. The self-defeating patient is also likely to be other-defeating.

Finally, before presenting some clinical material, I want to mention one other influence on my recent thinking about masochism—namely, Lacan's notion of *jouissance* (1959–1960). The patient's attachment to his symptoms is one of the most striking phenomena in masochism. One of Freud's most persuasive points was that the patient comes to you for help, and then fights you when you attempt to remove his symptoms. Simple translation of *jouissance* into such terms as enjoyment or satisfaction is misleading: *jouissance* involves a perverse pleasure in pain linked to the individual's repeated failure to obtain the forbidden pleasure associated with desired transgressions, oedipal or otherwise. Hence symptoms may unconsciously be regarded by the patient as treasures, sources of secret enjoyment (Zizek, 2008). One might even say that the patient's meaning and the patient's organization of self depends on the symptoms.

THE CASE OF MR. L

Mr. L was thirty-four years old when he came to analysis. Although reasonably successful in his profession, he did not experience enjoyment from his work or from his relationships with others. He spent many hours in the analysis focusing on his eleven-year marriage and the ways that his wife mistreated him. Here are the opening associations of a typical session: "I got home from work, and no sooner had I gotten in the door than Muriel started bitching at me. She told me I was inconsiderate because I had made the kids and her wait to eat dinner by coming home so late. She told me that I didn't know what it was like to keep two kids content and occupied while waiting for the other parent to come home. During dinner, it continued. She told me that I didn't do anything around the house to help her. She complained that all I do is watch TV instead of helping my son with his homework in the evenings. She said I tune her out when she talks to me. It went on and on. Finally, I told her I'd be glad to leave if she wants to get another husband. That comment infuriated her. She hurled the plate of pasta at me. It hit me in the head. The pasta fell on the floor, and both the kids started crying. I got down on the floor, picked up all the fragments of the plate so the kids wouldn't get cut, and then I cleaned up the pasta. I had no appetite after that so I walked out the back door and sat out in the yard. As I stared into the night, I thought of how much I hated my life and hated myself."

All of this was said with an air of resignation that this kind of interaction was a veritable certainty, a fated event each night that was etched in the granite of fate, so that analysis wouldn't really help any of it. I soon became another persecutor who failed to meet his needs. He struck me as both entitled and self-loathing at the same time, a good illustration of the mixture of narcissism and masochism described by Arnold Cooper (1993). After about a year of analysis, things came to a head around a request to change an hour. Because of a scheduling conflict he had with his one o'clock session on Monday, Mr. L asked me if I would be willing to see him in the late afternoon on Mondays. Since he had a work obligation that could not be changed, I told him I would look into my schedule and see what I could do. Four weeks later, I was able to free up the four o'clock hour on Monday. When I began a session with that announcement, he responded by saying that he no longer wished to change. He said that it had taken me so long to respond to his request that he had made some shifts at work that allowed him to continue coming at one. I was exasperated because I had already arranged for another patient to take that hour on Mondays.

With no more than a feeble effort to hide my irritation, I said to him: "I thought we had an understanding that I would attempt to change the hour, just as you requested." He replied: "I waited for weeks, and you did nothing, so I gave up. I think it's presumptuous of you to go ahead and change the hour weeks after I requested it." I retorted that I was simply honoring my agreement with him. He declared that it was no longer an agreement. I was quietly fuming at this point. I felt that I had gone to a great deal of trouble to accommodate him and that he was being completely unappreciative. I had become the masochist to his sadist. I suggested to him that this was a situation typical of others he described to me in which he not only found it difficult to express appreciation for efforts to accommodate him, but also seemed downright angry about them.

His response was telling: "You're right. I feel I'm entitled to treat others like shit and then be treated fairly. It's unjust. I know it's related to negative feelings I have about the analysis. I want to live in a world where no rules apply. I think I don't really want to be helped. I don't want to be in a position to be grateful. I am greedy and selfish. I'm a taker, not a giver. It's my goal to get you angry. I know I antagonize my wife and my colleagues in the same way."

I acknowledged that indeed he had made me angry, and I wondered with him what he got out of producing this response in others. He clarified it for me: "I don't want to feel indebted to others or feel helped because it makes me feel inadequate. I also kind of torment you. I imagine you're thinking: "For all this time I've helped this guy, and he never appreciates it." I know I do that to my wife. I'm hooked on torture."

After Mr. L left my office, I found myself frozen in my chair, feeling defeated, and indeed thinking that he was totally unappreciative of my efforts. I had a variety of retaliatory fantasies. I would simply shut down and stop trying to help him, forcing him to do all the work. Two could play at this game of medieval torture. Alternatively, I could aggressively interpret his contempt and point out that in defeating me he condemns himself to a life of misery from torturing others. Then I recognized, of course, that such a life might give him great pleasure. That night as I drove home, I thought to myself: "Just wait until the next time he wants to change an hour. I can be just as uncooperative as he can."

Mr. L came to the next session and told me about a conversation with his wife. She had asked him if analysis was helping him. He responded: "Gabbard thinks it helps me." He then told me that his wife had a message for me—namely, that it wasn't helping and that he was still nasty towards her. He went on to say: "I don't think you appreciate what I have to go through at home." I said to him that since he felt unappreciated by me, I wondered if he attempted to make me feel unappreciated by him. He then fell sound asleep.

In the course of his analysis, Mr. L frequently slept for substantial periods. I often felt a sense of exasperation that the analysis meant so little to him that it wasn't worth staying awake for. He once informed me that analysis was useful because my couch was comfortable to sleep on. Sometimes I was frankly relieved to have a break from him. At other times I felt his sleeping was a continued form of torment in which I had to masochistically endure him. He once woke up on the couch and said: "I guess I'm doing this to irritate you. It's a form of retaliation. You do something to me. I do something to you. My fantasy is that while I sleep, you are becoming increasingly enraged. I imagine that you will wake me up and throw me out of the office."

I interpreted to him: "In that scenario, I'm the angry one while you're simply the victim of my anger." He responded: "It's ingrained in my character to reject all responsibility for my own anger. I'll do anything to avoid making an active decision to get up and leave. I'd much rather have you throw me out."

I replied: "Of course, either way the analysis would be interrupted, and we would no longer be working together." Mr. L reflected for a moment and said: "I'm hooked on making people miserable. I have this fantasy that you want me to change, so I'm going to thwart your efforts. I used to think you needed me to graduate because you were a student. But then I heard from a friend of mine that you're a regular analyst who isn't in training. Still, I don't want to give up any power over you. Basically, I don't want to change. I know that you are invested in changing me, though. I see that book on your shelf, *The Treatment of Emotional Disorders*, and I realized that I misread it yesterday. I thought it said *The Treasury of Emotional Disorders*. I think I treasure and hold on to all my problems."

I suggested to Mr. L that his fantasy of hanging on to his problems and never changing also served another purpose: "If you succeed in thwarting my efforts and never changing, you can then go on indefinitely tormenting me. We'll be together forever."

My acknowledgement of his yearning for connectedness helped Mr. L become more reflective: "To give up this mode of interacting with people is to be disconnected and alone," he said. Here we can see one of the major themes of relational masochism — it's better to have a bad object than no object at all. Mr. L continued: "My parents always had the belief that I could do anything I wanted. I refused to follow through on what they wanted of me. I've had this intense love-hate relationship with them where they tried so hard to get me to live up to my potential. I got pleasure out of digging in my heels and refusing to do what they wanted."

I observed that this pattern of behavior maintained an intense bond with them. Mr. L went on: "I know. But you have to understand that my dad would often completely ignore me. You think my sleeping is bad? You should have seen him. He used to sleep all the time, and it absolutely infuriated me. I used to say in a loud voice, 'Would you wake up?' He'd say, 'Leave me alone! I work all day!' Then he'd snore, which would make me even more furious."

As I listened, I began to understand that Mr. L in his own way was unconsciously re-creating his experience with his father so that I could gain some firsthand appreciation of what he experienced. In addition, of course, Mr. L was telling me that I meant a great deal to him and that he did not want to lose our relationship. As he continued in this vein, he elaborated on this very notion: "I'm indebted to people because I can torment them and stay connected to them. My life has been dedicated to disappointing others. Failure is success. I'm perfectly willing to sacrifice myself to thwart others. I get no other comparable joy in my life. If I ever change as a result of analysis, I would only want to change after the grave—and that's how I think of termination—like death. I don't want you to have any satisfaction. Like my parents—they've done all this work and they get no pleasure. I imagine if I don't change and don't express my gratitude, you'll just keep thinking and worrying about me, even after my termination. You'll never get over me."

As I reflected on my own contributions to this two-person interaction, I realized that my bitterness led me to speak to him with a tone that undoubtedly sounded critical at times. Repeating the scenario that occurred with his parents, he sensed that I wanted him to fall in line with my expectations, and he derived great pleasure from digging in his heels and defeating me. I had failed to appreciate that he was trying to communicate to me that he was doing the analysis in the way he *had* to do it, and that my failure fed his own developmental difficulties in feeling appreciated or recognized.

As we moved towards termination, he spoke of his envy and competitiveness more. He said in the closing months of the analysis: "I should feel good at how patient you've been with me and how much I've gotten out of it, but I just can't acknowledge it. I see all the books on your shelf. I notice one by Winnicott. I've heard of him, and I think that I should have read that also. I want to read everything you've read, in part to compete with you, but in part so we'll stay connected. My fear of being alone comes up as I talk about terminating. I'll probably make the decision to stop being miserable after you're not around anymore. I've really learned a lot in here. I'm beginning to understand that that was the point of it all. I have very deep affection for you."

DISCUSSION

In this fragment of an analysis, one can see the multiple determinants of masochism at work. In the transference Mr. L re-created the "bad enough object" that fended off feelings of separation, loneliness and abandonment. Indeed, a bad object was much better than none at all. This re-creation also enabled him to work through longstanding negative interactions with his father from childhood in which he and I would alternate in who was the sadist/aggressor and who was the masochist/victim. The theme of ominipotence and narcissism was also embedded in his character structure. He presented himself as a Christ-like figure who was humiliated and unappreciated by his wife, enduring the slings and arrows of outrageous persecution by her. In the transference he felt entitled to special recognition from me for his heroic survival of such mistreatment. He also used his self-criticism to fend off attacks from the analyst.

Lacan's notion of *jouissance* is also relevant to this case. His masochistic suffering was a core part of his self-organization. In order to preserve his symptoms, Mr. L had to fend off the analyst's efforts to help. In his misreading of the textbook on my shelf, he revealed that his problems were his treasures, which he enjoyed in a perverse way. In his omnipotence fantasy, his preservation of his problems would result in hanging on to me forever in an unchanging and unending way.

Envy and competitiveness were also at play. He could not tolerate the idea that I had something to offer him that he lacked himself. He was willing to bring himself down to thwart me. In this regard, revenge was a powerful motivator in Mr. L. He bitterly resented the way his parents used him as an extension of their own narcissism and wanted him to succeed to make them look good. The Yiddish term *naches* refers to the pleasure that parents take in their children's successes. Mr. L was triumphant in depriving his parents of that pleasure and thus taking revenge on them. In the transference, this theme was also re-enacted as he waited until after termination to make the real changes.

Mr. L's striving to create miserable situations in which he was mistreated by others, whether his wife or his analyst, was clearly better than something else. It was better than following a script that his parents had written for him—a scenario in which he would be the star of the family and THEY would steal his thunder by taking all the credit for his accomplishments while blaming HIM for any failures that occurred. The sadistic triumph of defying their programming, embarrassing them and depriving them of the pleasure of being the good son they wanted was far better than leading a good life.

CONCLUSION

The analytic clinician must look for a variety of threads in the patient material that weave the tapestry of masochism. Determinants from different developmental levels will regularly be found. Moreover, masochistic patients will generally demonstrate that they are adept at tormenting others in addition to tormenting the self. Analysts treating these patients need to systematically interpret the sadistic and hostile themes in the patient's unconscious often masked by masochistic submission. Much of the pleasure of the masochistic patient may be derived from taking revenge on the parents by defying their expectations. Patients can be helped considerably if they see that in reality they are undermining themselves when they strive to defeat or sabotage their parents' plan for them.

REFERENCES

Bion, W. R. (1959). Attacks on linking. In *Second Thoughts*. New York: Aronson, 1967, 93–109.

Bromberg, P. M. (1996). Hysteria, dissociation, and the cure of Emmy von N revisited. *Psychoanalytic Dialogues* 6: 55–71.

Cooper, A. (1993). Psychotherapeutic approaches to masochism. *Journal of Psychotherapy Practice and Research* 2: 51–63.

Cooper, S. H. (2010). Self-criticism and unconscious grandiosity: Transference-countertransference dimensions. *International Journal of Psychoanalysis* 91: 1115–36.

Fenichel O. (1945). *The Psychoanalytic Theory of the Neuroses*. New York: International Universities Press.

Gabbard, G. O. (1996). *Love and Hate in the Analytic Setting*. Northvale, NJ: Jason Aronson.

——— (2000). On gratitude and gratification. *Journal of the American Psychoanalytic Association* 48: 697–716.

Gabbard, G. O., and Lester, E. P. (2003). *Boundaries and Boundary Violations in Psychoanalysis*. Washington, D.C.: American Psychiatric Press.

Klein, M. (1957). Envy and gratitude. In *The Writings of Melanie Klein: Vol. 3. Envy and Gratitude and Other Works, 1946–1963*. New York: Free Press, 1975, 176–235.

Lacan, J. (1959–1960). *The Seminar: Book VII: The Ethics of Psychoanalysis, 1959–60*, translated by Dennis Porter, notes by Dennis Porter. London: Routledge, 1992.

Rosen, I. R. (1993). Relational masochism: The search for a bad-enough object. Presented to the Topeka Psychoanalytic Society, January 21.

Zizek, S. (2008). *Enjoy Your Symptom!* London: Routledge, 2008.

SEVEN

Self-Abuse and Suicidality: Clinical Manifestations of Chronic Narcissistic Rage

Anna Ornstein, MD

Sally, a twenty-three-year-old college student, in twice weekly psycho-therapy, frequently discussed an elaborate fantasy of killing herself and having all her friends who had mistreated her go to the funeral and finally feel guilt and remorse about how they had emotionally brutalized her to the point where she had been driven to end her life. This fantasy, and her rage in response to actual or imagined insults, would qualify Sally a place among a cluster of patients who, depending on their thera-pists' theoretical orientation, would receive the diagnosis either of maso-chistic or borderline personality disorder.

The psychoanalytic view of sadomasochism has undergone many changes in the history of psychoanalysis. As long as the outstanding subjective experience included suffering, a variety of clinical pictures have been included into this diagnostic category. Any precision or consis-tency in labeling has been difficult because various clinical descriptions have been interpreted with the help of a variety of theoretical constructs and given a variety of psychological meanings. Maleson (1984) reviewed the shifting, often obscure and ambiguous interpretations of masochism and explored the possible resolution of this diagnostic and theoretical confusion. He recommended that we "accept and legitimize the common usage of masochism as a term loosely denoting phenomena in which suffering, submission, or defeat are especially prominent or tenacious, and simply seem necessary, 'driven,' or in some way self-induced in the judgment of the analyst" (Maleson, 1984). Others (Simons, 1987; Kernberg 1988) attempted to bring organization and clarity to the differing conceptualizations by distinguishing two groups in the manifest clinical picture: "depressive-masochism" and "sadomasochism." In the latter, there appears to be less conflict in expressing sadism *directly* than in the former. Glick and Meyers (1988), in their review of the psychoanalytic literature, made an effort to disentangle the relationship between overt sexual masochism on the one hand and characterological (or moral) masochism, on the other. These authors came to the conclusion that no sharp delineation could be made; there appears to be a continuum between these two forms of masochism.

Since metapsychological considerations concern themselves with the *origin* of this personality disorder, they have greater clinical significance for psychoanalysis than do diagnoses on the clinical, manifest level. The function of suffering as the main feature of masochism was understood and interpreted in keeping with the analyst's theoretical orientation: it was conceptualized either as arising in relation to drive vicissitudes (Brenner, 1959; Loewenstein, 1957) or as an ego defense and/or disturbed early object relationships (Berliner, 1947; Menaker, 1953; Bernstein, 1957). Those who remained faithful to Freud's original formulation explained the motive for the pain and suffering as a *condition* for the attainment of pleasure (Freud, 1905, 1915; Reich, 1933; Reik, 1941), a view that preserved the pleasure principle as an important aspect of the libido theory. Ego psychology viewed masochism as a compromise formation where unconscious guilt is supposed to play a particularly important role by permitting, simultaneously, gratification and punishment for forbidden incestuous sexual wishes.

It is of significance that while ego psychology adhered to the pathogenic significance of drive-related fantasies, psychoanalysts, at the same time, took note of the frequency with which patients suffering from this disorder had been traumatized in their childhoods: "It is now generally assumed from the reports of numerous writers that the masochist had undergone a most considerable degree of traumatization in very early life. With great frequency, we uncover severe periods of emotional deprivation, absence of loving care of the parents" (Socarides, 1958, p. 588).

Many features associated with sadomasochism are found in the general, non-clinical population. In his extensive discussion of the subject, Grossman (1986) stated: "At present, there is general agreement that there are phenomena deserving to be called masochism or masochistic to be found in normal people as well as in people with a variety of pathological syndrome" (p. 382).

Beginning in the 1970s and 1980s following Kohut's publications on narcissism (1966, 1968, 1971, 1972, 1978), a number of papers appeared (Stolorow, 1975; Fischer, 1981) drawing attention to the close connection between masochism and narcissism. Stolorow (1975) argued that both masochism and sadism affect the narcissistic sector of the personality: "It is safe to assume that early, pre-oedipal traumata implicated in the origins of severe masochism would also leave marking on the narcissistic sector by interfering with the development of a cohesive and stable self-represetentation" (p. 442). Cooper, who considered pre-oedipal traumatic experiences to be of great significance, suggested that the clinical picture in these cases is dominated by "masochistic-narcissistic defenses" where "the aim is not a reunion with a loving mother, but a fantasized control over a cruel and damaging mother," as reported by Fischer (1981, p. 677).

CLINICAL EXAMPLE

In everyday practice, psychoanalysts and psychoanalytically oriented psychotherapists do not concern themselves with descriptive diagnoses. The outstanding features of patients' personalities emerge in the course of treatment and are highlighted by the nature of the transference. Only in the course of psychotherapy or analysis can we recognize the sources of the disorder. In addition, as I indicated earlier, what a clinician may consider to be the origin of this disorder, depends on his/her theoretical orientation. The following clinical report was guided by psychoanalytic self psychology. The condensed report of a four year treatment is focused on the patient's transferences and will include samples of the therapeutic dialogue[1] that I consider to have been decisive in the therapeutic results the patient was able to achieve.

Dr. White came to see me because he feared that his wife would soon ask him to leave because he has not been able to be a husband to her nor a father to their eight-year-old daughter and four-year-old son. Dr. White, a forty-five-year-old research scientist, whose weekly psychotherapy was converted to psychoanalysis after two years, had entertained fantasies similar to Sally's. He kept a vial of a toxic substance in his drawer; when he felt particularly desperate, he found solace in knowing that he could put an end to his mental anguish anytime he wanted. He would then imagine how remorseful his wife would be for never putting her arms around him and never telling him that she loved him.

The patient was a short, very slightly built man. His pale, heavily lined forehead and neatly trimmed graying beard were in sharp contrast to his very lean body and extremities which looked as if they belonged to a twelve-year-old boy rather than to a forty-five-year-old man. He had all the symptoms associated with a severe case of anorexia, except that of a distorted body image: he felt thin and was fully aware of the dangers involved in keeping his weight barely above acceptable limits. He also engaged in lengthy exercises every day; he set his alarm for 2:30 a.m. but frequently got up before that in order to complete the time-consuming routine of weight lifting and running. With his near starvation diet, strenuous exercises and his chronic sleep deprivation, he felt exhausted all the time. In relation to food or rest, he felt compelled to deprive himself of anything that could potentially give him pleasure.

The patient's own parents divorced before he was three years old; he had no memory of his mother. He knew that his mother was alcoholic and that, after the divorce, his father did not permit her to visit him and his two years younger sister. It was in the course of his analysis that my patient learned from his father that he was repeatedly hospitalized for broken bones, bruises over his body and burns on his hands and feet; injuries that his mother had inflicted on him. His father, also a scientist, had extremely high standards for the children's behavior and raised them with strict puritanical methods. Dr. White was always an A student but could not recall having ever felt satisfaction or that his father ever expressed satisfaction with him or with his accomplishments. He was always left with the feeling that he could have done better. He was a chubby child and his father, in order to teach him good eating habits and self-restraint, did not allow him to enter the kitchen before going to school. Instead, he would bring the patient an orange for breakfast to his room. His father also stressed the importance of physical activities, and the patient became a successful long-distance runner which earned him several trophies. In spite of the fact that he has been able to secure prestigious and large grants over the years, he worried that he will be asked to leave his current job because he did not meet the high standards of the institution where he worked.

The patient could not recall any time when he was able to ask for physical or emotional comfort freely and directly. He no longer experienced the longing for close emotional contact in its original form; this was now mixed with shame and it found expression in a behavior pattern in which he presented himself in a pitiful, sorrowful way: he walked with his shoulders hunched, frequently emitting a deep sigh and whenever he had the opportunity, he would make degrading remarks about himself or about his work. Entering my office, he would regularly emit an audible sigh and lower himself into the chair as if that would be too much of an exertion. I understood this behavior pattern as "the masochist's bid for affection," a pattern of behavior in which *sadism is expressed indirectly* by making others, his current transference objects, feel guilty for his mental suffering (Berliner, 1958). Expectedly, such behavior does not produce compassion. Rather, it is experienced as an accusation for one's suffering and an unspoken demand for reparation. Instead of eliciting compassion, people who witness it, turn away from such guilt-creating demand. In the course of Dr. White's treatment, we came to refer to this as "feel-sorry-for-me" behavior.

Because of this indirect communication of displaced rage, Dr. White suffered repeated rejections by the very people whose accepting and validating responses he craved and needed most urgently. Eventually, he realized that even when others were responsive to his indirect appeals for emotional comfort, he could not reciprocate this; while he had an enormous need for affection, he could neither receive nor reciprocate it. For my patient, the "feel-sorry-for-me" behavior constituted the final common pathway, a symptomatic behavior with multiple functions. Though derived from a very different theoretical perspective, my view of this masochistic behavior pattern is similar to one stated by Brenman (1952) who, with the thorough study of a single case, maintained that masochism serves multiple functions and any one explanation falls short of understanding this complex clinical picture.

For Dr. White, the longing for a caring and accepting response had become associated not only with rage and shame but also with jealousy and envy of those whom he experienced as receiving attention while he felt excluded or dismissed. In his jealous rages he would humiliate and verbally abuse his four-year-old son, the recipient of his wife's affection. The patient was convinced that it was the birth of this child that "pushed me over the brink," and he dated his depression, his suicidality and the anorexia to the birth of his now four-year-old son. He told me of an episode when he literally tore the child away from his mother because he was touching her breast. It appears that his son touching his wife's breast had activated an intense need for physical comfort and intimacy. Once the need for the hug and the touch were activated so was his sense of frustration that caused him either to strike out impulsively or to withdraw in hurt and anger. The angry and guilt-provoking retreat would say in essence: "You are depriving me, you are a bad, withholding mother and even if you tried to give to me, I know it will not be enough . . . or not *exactly* what I need."

After a rage outburst at his son, Dr. White would experience intense shame, and he would become acutely suicidal. In order to protect himself as well as his family from his rage outbursts and the shame and guilt that would follow, Dr. White frequently remained at work late at night and would leave the house before the children woke up in the morning. He rarely participated in family activities and in fear that his fantasy of a "perfect holiday" would not be fulfilled, he would take on extra assignments and would stay at work during the holidays. At these times he would be filled with self-pity and a renewed determination to kill himself before the next major holiday.

During his treatment, the patient did not become acutely suicidal. However, I regarded his anorexia as a form of suicide. Schneidman (1976) considered anorexia, bulimia, self-cutting, and alcohol and drug addictions as expressions of chronic suicidality and distinguished these from acute suicide which, in his view, only lasts a few hours. Suicidality appears to be a compromise between the wish to die and the ongoing effort to extract a response from the environment that could save the sufferer from mental agony. Chronic suicidality may or may not be associated with a major psychiatric illness such as schizophrenia, depression, or a severe personality disorder. In my patient, I considered the suicidality to be an aspect of his sadomasochistic personality organization.

Because of the severity of his depression and the suicide risk, the patient was put on an anti-depressant which, after some time, began to relieve his depression. However, the medication did not alter the sadomasochistic behavior pattern and had only minimal effect on the anorexia; the patient continued to feel emotionally isolated and chronically enraged.

Since his wife had become Dr. White's most important transference object, he was strongly motivated to display the "feel-sorry-for-me" behavior in her presence. For example, one day when he was particularly successful at work and was looking forward to going home in a reasonably good mood, he realized that as he was nearing his home he became increasingly more irritable and depressed. By the time he reached the house, he convinced himself that the good feelings of the day were nothing but an illusion. He realized then, he said to me, that: "presenting myself as a failure is the best way for me to communicate my despair. . . . I am afraid she [wife] will see me feeling good."

The couple had not shared a bedroom since the birth of their second child. Whenever his wife approached him physically, he always found a reason to withdraw from her. He finally asked me: "Why can't I accept her efforts to comfort me?" I thought that with this question we had achieved our first therepeutic aim: the patient had become introspective. I felt encouraged and offered a rather comprehensive interpretive comment. I said that it seems that his wife had become a mother to him who, he felt, ought to make up for what he did not get from his own mother. When she failed in this, this was a repetition of his childhood experiences and he would become enraged at her. I said that at his age, it is difficult to consider that his behavior may have more to do with the past than with the present. My comments were met with a deep sigh and a long silence. Before he left, the patient commented that he will have to think about what I had just said. The next day, he told me that he considered my comments and what I said made him feel worse rather than better; he now had to realize how childish his behavior has been and how unreasonable he is. I said that I could understand that it is easier for me than for him to consider that he wished his wife would be the mother he never had, to get from her what his mother never gave him: love and tenderness. Pulling his head deep into his chest, the patient remained silent for the rest of the hour.

In the next phase of treatment, the close examination of his relationship with his wife became the focus of our therapeutic dialogue. He wondered again and again why he could not accept her efforts to comfort him. I repeated my earlier comment and added that this most likely related to the anger he experienced but could not express as a child. As much as he needs to be comforted now, he cannot accept this from his wife because, in his mind, she is also the "bad mother" on whom he feels compelled to take revenge. This made sense to the patient as he was familiar with his efforts to find fault with her and how angry he would get when she did not do *exactly* what he expected from her. It seems to me, I said, that his greatest dilemma now is that he craves attention and caring, but cannot accept it—instead, he feels repeatedly frustrated and enraged.

The exploration of the nature of his relationship to his wife took us back to the onset of his difficulties: the birth of his son. In response to my comments, Dr. White would make barely audible comments about the unreasonableness of his behavior and said that he could never accept such childish feelings in himself. In an effort to help him accept his "childish" feelings, I said that I could see how after the birth of his son, the longing for unconditional acceptance, love, and attention had become more imperative. I said I could well understand that when these were not forthcoming and not exactly the way he needed them, he would become frustrated and enraged. Looking at his behavior with a cool head after such episodes, he would be filled with shame and remorse. Dr. White remembered then that he had similar problems after the birth of his daughter but was able to overcome them.

The transference nature of his relationship with his wife was not difficult to detect: his infantile longings and the associated frustrations and rage were readily activated by her relationship with their infant son. However, since his hopes and expectations in relation to me appeared only in highly disguised forms, his transferences toward me were more difficult to identify.

The transferences that patients develop in relation to their analysts and other important people in their lives depend on the responses they receive in these different relationships. As long as analysts maintain an empathic listening perspective, the fate of the transference that emerges in an analytic relationship will be very different from the one that emerges in other intimate relationships. Analysts listening empathically aim at understanding, and by offering empathic interpretive comments are accepting of their patients' transference needs. A similar empathic attitude and response, however, is not likely to greet the patient in other important relationships. There, the defensively disguised childhood developmental need for unconditional acceptance or for an enthusiastic response is either not recognized or outright rejected. Under these circumstances, relationships in the patient's adult life may become true repetitions of the original traumatic ones and lifelong, symptomatic behavior patterns persist and become fortified. Experiencing the imperative nature of their transference needs, patients become oblivious to the way in which they are experienced by others; rather than securing positive self-object responses, with their guilt-provoking behavior, they provoke renewed rejections. In other words, in non-therapeutic relationships, patients are likely to be frustrated in their transference expectations that lead to the escalation of their demands, to mutual recriminations and retaliations; no wonder that such relationships do not facilitate experiencing others as potentially new selfobjects (Ornstein, 1990).

This does not mean that repetitions of old behavior do not occur in empathically conducted treatment. When patients finally become engaged in treatment, they might provoke some of the most insidious and difficult to overcome countertransference problems: perceiving the demand for perfect responsiveness and the rage whenever this is being frustrated, analysts may unconsciously pull back from such demands and subsequent rage reactions. Protracted transference-countertransference entanglements make the maintenance of an empathic listening perspective extremely challenging and analysts may find themselves rejecting their patients in subtle ways, unwittingly repeating the patient's original trauma. No other group of patients can end up in a hopeless impasse in treatment as frequently as does this group of patients.

The following set of associations helped us understand what Dr. White needed from me, his analyst. He began an hour by telling me a story he heard on the radio about a man describing the sexual experiences of another person. He thought at first that it was a gay man describing the sexual experience of another man. Then he realized that the man was talking about the sexual experiences of a woman. He wondered how a man could know anything about the sexual experience of a woman. I said though I could not be sure, but I did have an idea why these stories had come to his mind now and why he may have wanted to tell me about them. I thought these stories had to do with the same question he raised before when he told me about a poem with the refrain: "nobody can understand the suffering of his fellowman." I said that it has been very important for him, I said that others knew how he felt, as if his painful feelings would be easier to bear by sharing them. I continued: "But then he may have wondered: could anyone really know how he felt? Could I know the depth of his suffering? After all, my life experiences had to be different from his." "Yes," he said, "I often wondered about that." As a matter of fact, he often worried that should he doubt my understanding and appreciation of how much he is suffering emotionally, then, in our relationship too, he may feel compelled to resort to something drastic in order to convince me about the depth of his misery. Imagining that I would become upset and distraught upon hearing about his suicide, he felt elated. That made him wonder: could he actually go that far to assure that I knew the extent of his mental anguish? He thought about this the other day and realized that though I had never discussed with him his suicidal intent directly, or tried to talk him out of it, he could not be sure if I could understand what life was like for him. He recalled that, though he did not like my explanation for his reasons for trying to get attention from his wife with his "feel-sorry-for-me" behavior, it gave him hope that his behavior made sense to me, that I knew *how he felt*. "You are my last hope that what I feel can be known," he said. "Otherwise, being miserable is my 'lifeline' to others."

Conversations of this nature made me hopeful. My interpretive comments regarding his complex (transference) relationship with his wife appeared not to be as important to him as the fact that his contradictory feelings toward her made sense to me. Dr. White knew that I understood how he felt: desperately needing attention and love but unable to receive and reciprocate it because he was too angry too much of the time. He repeated what he had told me before, namely that the only thing that could save him would be to know that what he felt made sense and that it could be understood. In considering therapeutic action in psychoanalysis, we (Ornstein, 1992; Ornstein and Ornstein, 1996) had found repeatedly that feeling understood constitutes one of the most important elements in the healing process. Conveying understanding and acceptance is what Winnicott (1965) meant when he said: "Holding the patient often takes the form of conveying *in words* at the appropriate moment something that shows that *the analyst knows and understands the deepest anxiety that is being experienced*" (p. 240, italics added). Once understood, he could share his feelings, and the sense of isolation he felt most of his life could be lessened, at least in relationship to me. He said that feeling that his "crazy" behavior made sense to me made him feel that he is not alone in the world.

Following conversations of this nature, Dr. White began an hour by telling me that the day before he felt good. He went home at a reasonable hour and had dinner with his family, something he hadn't done for a long time; he did not run off to the basement to do his exercises as he usually had done. But now, he is already worried that his good feelings will not last; that tonight something may set him off, and once that happens, he will not be able to stop himself from repeating his old pattern: once he feels hurt, he will have to retaliate immediately or withdraw in fear of abusing his family.

While we made slow but steady progress in translating the "feel-sorry-for me" behavior into its multiple meanings, the anorexia and his commitment to strenuous exercises remained stubborn enactments of his sadomasochistic personality organization. Eventually, we found the key to our understanding of his fear of eating tasty and potentially nourishing food: this was the symptom that connected him most securely to his father. The father remained the one person in his life who was always pleased to hear from him but also the one who did not refrain from telling his son how to live his life. When his wife eventually suggested divorce, his father encouraged the patient to move out of their home right away.

The separation and divorce proved beneficial to the patient in totally unexpected ways. After he rented an empty apartment and tried to discourage the children from visiting him because "I don't even have a bed for you," the children, especially his son, insisted on visiting his father. The child told him that he would be willing to sleep on the floor so that he could see his father regularly. This was an unexpected gift: someone whom the patient had in many ways neglected, expressed a wish to be with him. At first, this was more than he could understand and accept, but the child was insistent. After a few sleep-overs, the child asked his father to take him to a baseball game. When the patient told me that rather than just sitting on the bench and feeling miserable, he joined in with the crowd in their enthusiastic response to the game, I realized that significant structural changes (for example, his ability not to respond instantaneously with rage when frustrated) must have taken place in the course of treatment that had been too subtle for me to register.

Similar to his earlier focus on his relationship with his wife, the patient now focused on his relationship with his children, especially with his son. Early in the treatment, Dr. White told me that because of his father's importance to him, his greatest desire was to become a good father but that his reaction to his son's birth made that impossible. At this time, I reminded him that he now had another chance; with his insistence to spend time with his father, his son made the feel-sorry-for-me behavior irrelevant. The child's genuine desire to be with his father had reached Dr. White in a way that my most carefully phrased interpretations could not. However, I believe that while my earlier interpretive comments prepared him for being able to feel loved and accepted by his children, his son reaching out to him proved to be the transformative experience he needed for his recovery. Recognizing the importance of his ability to experience enthusiasm and his ability to welcome and reciprocate his children's affection, I became more actively validating of these changes in him. His life circumstances and experiencing me as being well connected to his changing emotions ushered in a period of rapid improvement. Dr. White no longer considered the thought of suicide as a needed comfort; with increasing frequency, he enjoyed his work and spending time with his children. After he put on weight, he had become increasingly more physically and emotionally resilient. He eventually married a woman he knew from his workplace and who, he felt, was warm and affectionate with him. My own understanding was that he was now able to perceive and reciprocate the genuine affection of others. These changes determined the time of termination. The ideal time for termination, Kohut (1977) wrote, is when "the analysand's self has become firm, when it ceases to react to the loss of selfobjects with fragmentation, serious enfeeblement, or uncontrollable rage" (p. 138). In cases of severe self pathology when sadomasochistic behavior patterns are keeping a fragmented, suicidal self barely functional, termination is indicated when patients are able to utilize currently available selfobjects for the maintenance of their self-cohesion without resorting to habitual, pathological defense organizations.

After termination, I saw Dr. White with some frequency in the neighborhood where both of our offices were located. He no longer looked emaciated, and I was delighted to see him walking with a spring in his stride.

COMMENTS ON THE SELF PSYCHOLOGICAL
PERSPECTIVE OF SADOMASOCHISM

All psychoanalytic theories trace the origin of psychopathology to the patient's infancy and childhood and so does psychoanalytic self psychology. In self psychology, the origins of sadomasochism, as with other forms of personality disorders, are traced to *lived experiences* rather than to unconscious, drive-related fantasies. In this theoretical perspective, what determines health and illness from a developmental perspective is the way in which individual biology (temperament, genes, intellect, and special endowments) effects the organization of environmental experiences: infants are active organizers of their experiences. Present-day theory of pathogenesis has to consider a person's ability to summon necessary defenses (projection, denial, disavowal, externalization, identification, etc.) to safeguard self-cohesion. This has implications for the treatment process. Defensive operations and symptoms are not viewed here as having to be removed in order to expose an unacceptable truth related to sex and aggression; rather, they are recognized as necessary "strategies" to protect an enfeebled self from fragmentation.

The developmental theory of self psychology asserts that what is required during infancy for the building up of well functioning psychological structures are phase-appropriate merger experiences with the caretaker's selfobject functions such as the caretaker's calmness and soothing voice. The internalization of these caretaker functions is responsible for the development of the capacity to regulate tension and anxiety, to calm and soothe oneself. And it is the phase-appropriate recognition and validation (mirroring) of a child's growing capacities that transforms the infantile narcissistic structures (grandiosity and exhibitionism) into pride and pleasure in one's self and in one's activities; self-cohesion and self-esteem are gradually built by the caretakers' unambivalent responsiveness to the child's uniqueness and his/her accomplishments. The absence or faulty responses of these developmentally needed functions by caretakers lead to the persistence of infantile grandiosity in the adult psyche which explains the tenacity with which patients may cling to a sense of absolute perfection on the part of their environment. The failure of transformation of infantile narcissistic structures (grandiosity and exhibitionism) leaves the self devoid of vigor, aliveness and a reliable self-esteem regulatory system. Instead, patients suffer from a sense of emptiness and worthlessness; a self so riddled with defects and deficits lacks resilience and is extremely vulnerable to rejections to which patients react either with wholesale withdrawal or unforgiving rage. When physical abuse is added to this scenario, children—and later as adults—experience themselves as undeserving of love and having any pleasure in life.

Being deprived of legitimate developmentally needed merger and mirroring experiences and traumatic experiences such as physical, sexual, and verbal abuse create narcissistic rage which cannot be voiced in childhood because this could further threaten the precarious connection to a rejecting and abusive environment. In order to assure continued connection to the frustrating and/or abusive caretaker, infants and young children develop what Branchaft (2007) called "pathological accommodations" that function as protection "against intolerable pain and existential anxiety" (p. 667).

Adults may express repressed and/or disavowed chronic narcissistic rage either directly or indirectly: Sadistic behavior (unleashing the rage at the frustrating other with physical and/or verbal assault) expresses the rage directly; there can be no question regarding its intent and intensity. In masochistic behavior, rage finds expression in indirect ways. The unrelenting demand to right past wrongs may find a variety of behavioral expressions: an angry, chip-on-the-shoulder attitude, holding grudges and collecting injustices or a "feel-sorry-for-me" behavior, haughty withdrawal, writing people off, self-recrimination, and various degrees of depression. The indirectly expressed rage is a powerful accusation implying that one's mental anguish was carelessly or deliberately inflicted by the frustrating other (Berliner, 1958).

This observation by Berliner has been of particular importance to my own understanding of this complex personality disorder. In my view, it best explains the frequently observed phenomenon that humiliation and verbal and physical abuse suffered in childhood may find expression in adult life in insisting that current transference objects take responsibility for and redeem the narcissistic injuries of the past. Kohut's (1972) description of the imperative need for revenge by all who suffered narcissistic injury gives further credence to Berliner's observation:

> Narcissistic rage occurs in many forms, they all share, however, a specific psychological flavor which gives them a distinct position within a wide realm of human aggression. The need for revenge, for righting a wrong, for undoing a hurt by whatever means and a deeply anchored, unrelenting compulsion of all these aims, which gives no rest to those who suffered a narcissistic injury—these are the characteristic features of narcissistic rage in all its forms which sets it apart from other kinds of aggression. (pp. 637–38)

These theoretical considerations help us understand that while masochistic behaviors, in all their varied patterns, have multiple functions, two stand out among them. On the one hand, they make a *demand* on the environment for love and acceptance; on the other hand, anticipating the frustrations of their infantile needs, they are also *retaliatory* in nature: taking revenge on the offending "other" that holds the illusory promise of restituting an injured self.

Developmental conditions are not always as extreme as was the case in Dr. White's early life where the physical abuse by one parent (mother) was followed by conditional acceptance by the other (father). While many features of the patient's sadomasochism could be traced to the early, totally repressed abuses by his mother, his attachment to his rigid and exacting father had also played a significant role. When acceptance and appreciation are thus conditioned, the child grows up with a nagging sense of self-doubt; doubt in his intellectual and/or physical abilities and attractiveness. Though Dr. White was a much-appreciated research scientist, he never experienced a sense of satisfaction, pride or contentment in his achievements.

SUMMARY

The theoretical explication of a clinical example with the outstanding feature of mental suffering served to demonstrate the self psychological understanding of sadomasochism. The review of the clinical material included samples of the analytic interactions in order to demonstrate how the analyst's theoretical orientation guided her interventions. In this treatment, the interpretations of the patient's extra analytic transferences provided important clues to the understanding of the nature of the psychopathology, while his transference toward the analyst demonstrated that feeling understood is an essential aspect of the healing process. The patient's ability to experience enthusiasm and to receive and to reciprocate his childrens' love indicated structural changes. These changes found expression in his increasing ability to regulate tension: he could now reflect on his affective states so that he no longer became instantaneously enraged and be compelled to retaliate or to withdraw.

NOTE

1. A therapeutic dialogue is a form of conversation in which the analyst does not wait until all parts of a puzzle fall into place. Instead, the analyst offers his/her tentative interpretive comments throughout the treatment. This has several advantages over "empathic inquiry." It orients the patient to the way the therapist has heard him and offers him the opportunity to disagree or further elaborate on the analyst's under-

standing. Such a dialogue deepens the process without creating hard to manage resistances as unconscious and barely conscious aspects of the patient's behavior and attitude are gradually drawn into the dialogue (Ornstein and Ornstein, 1986, 1996).

REFERENCES

Berliner, B. (1947). On some psychodynamics of masochism. *Psychoanalytic Quarterly* 16: 459–71.

———— (1958). The role of object relations in moral masochism. *Psychoanalytic Quarterly* 27: 38–56.

Bernstein, I. (1957). The role of narcissism in moral masochism. *Psychoanalytic Quarterly* 26: 358–77.

Branchaft, B. (2007). Systems of pathological accommodations and change in analysis. *Psychoanalytic Psychology* 24: 667–87.

Brenner, C. (1959). The masochistic character: Genesis and treatment. *Journal of the American Psychoanalytic Association* 7: 197–226.

Brenman, M. (1952). On teasing and being teased; and the problem of moral masochism. *Psychoanalytic Study of the Child* 7: 264–85.

Cooper, A. M., and Sacks, M. H. (1991). Sadism and masochism in character disorder and resistance. *Journal of the American Psychoanalytic Association* 39: 215–26

Fischer, N. (1981). Masochism: Current concepts. *Journal of the American Psychoanalytic Association* 29: 673–88.

Freud, S. (1905). Three essays on the theory of sexuality. *Standard Edition* 7: 123–246.

———— (1915). Instincts and their vicissitudes. *Standard Edition* 14: 109–40.

Glick, R., and Myers, D. (1988). *Masochism*. Hillsdale, NJ: Analytic Press.

Grossman, W. (1986). Notes on masochism: A discussion of the history and development of a psychoanalytic concept. *Psychoanalytic Quarterly* 60: 379–413.

Kernberg, O. F. (1988). Clinical dimensions of masochism. *Journal of the American Psychoanalytic Association* 36: 1005–29.

Kohut, H. (1966). Forms and transformations of narcissism. *Journal of the American Psychoanalytic Association* 14: 243–72. (Also in *Search for the Self* 1, ed. P. Ornstein, 427–75.)

———— (1968). The psychoanalytic treatment of narcissistic personality disorder—Outline of a systematic approach. *Psychoanalytic Study of the Child* 23: 86–113. (Also in *Search for the Self* 1, ed. P. Ornstein, 477–509.)

———— (1971). *The Analysis of the Self*. New York: International Universities Press.

———— (1972). Thoughts on narcissism and narcissistic rage. *Psychoanalytic Study of the Child* 27: 360–400.

———— (1977). *The Restoration of the Self*. New York: International Universities Press.

Loewenstein, R. (1957). A contribution to the psychoanalytic theory of masochism. *Journal of the American Psychoanalytic Association* 5: 197–234.

Maleson, F. (1984). The multiple meanings of masochism in psychoanalytic discourse. *Journal of the American Psychoanalytic Association* 32: 325–56.

Menaker, E. (1953). Masochism—A defense reaction of the ego. *Psychoanalytic Quarterly* 22: 205–20.

Ornstein, A. (1990). Selfobject transferences and the process of working through. *Progress in Self Psychology*. Hillsdale, NJ: Analytic Press.

———— (1992). The curative fantasy and psychic recovery. *Journal of Psychotherapy Practice and Research* 1: 16–28.

Ornstein, A., and Ornstein, P. H. (1986). Empathy and the therapeutic dialogue. *The Lydia Rappaport lecture Series* (1984), Smith School of Social Work, Northampton, MA.

———— (1996). Speaking in the interpretive mode and feeling understood: Crucial aspects of the therapeutic action in psychoanalysis. In *Understanding Therapeutic Ac-*

tion: Psychoanalytic Concepts of Cure, ed. L. E. Lifson. Hillsdale, NJ: Analytic Press, 87–101.

Reich, W. (1933). *Character Analysis*. New York: Orgon Institute Press, 1945.

Reik, T. (1941). *Masochism in Modern Man*. New York: Farrar & Reinhart.

Schneidman, E. S. (1976). The components of suicide. *Psychiatric Annals* 6: 51–66.

Simons, R. C. (1987). Psychoanalytic contributions to psychiatric nosology: Forms of masochistic behavior. *Journal of the American Psychoanalytic Association* 35: 583–608.

Socarides, C. W. (1958). The function of moral masochism: With special reference to the defence processes. *International Journal of Psychoanalysis* 39: 587–97.

Stolorow, R. D. (1975). The narcissistic function of masochism (and sadism). *International Journal of Psychoanalysis* 56: 441–48.

Winnicott, D. (1965). *The Maturational Processes and the Facilitating Environment*. London: Hogarth Press.

EIGHT

Varieties of Masochistic Experience: Modes of Analytic Relating

Henry Markman, MD

> It's very hard for our patients to find it possible to abandon such terrible delights for the uncertain pleasures of real relationships. . . . The masochistic state, then has a hold on the patient that is much stronger than the pull toward human relationships.
>
> —Betty Joseph, 1982, p. 456

I do not think there is anything more enigmatic for the analyst, and important to understand, than the drive toward suffering and destructiveness, often self-destructiveness—a turning away from life and opportunity toward pain and desolation. The intensity of this drive often makes analysis difficult and at times impossible, and accounts for impasses, negative therapeutic reactions and failed and abandoned treatments. Bearing the countertransference reactions in working with highly masochistic patients is a difficult task. Sadomasochistic enactments are common. The analysis of masochistic destructiveness is challenging and raises difficult technical issues regarding ways of listening and interpreting. I am inclined to think that some of the major theoretical and clinical innovations in psychoanalysis—certainly in Sigmund Freud's work—resulted from the clinical encounters with masochistic patients and the drive toward destructiveness. For example, the transition from libido theory to object relations theory and the structural theory in papers such as "Mourning and Melancholia" (1917), "A Child is Being Beaten" (1919), "Beyond the Pleasure Principle" (1920), "The Economic Problem of Masochism" (1924), and "On Transience" (1916) were for Freud spurred on by unsuccessful treatments, the need for longer treatments, and the horror of the Great War. The destructive aspect of the superego became a central concept in understanding masochistic and neurotic suffering. This aspect of Freud's theory inspired Melanie Klein's innovations, and eventually, the analytic ideas I will present today. For Klein, the conflict shifted from superego prohibitions and persecution toward unacceptable wishes, to the conflict between life instincts (loving) and the pull toward death and destructiveness.

My title is meant to convey the complexity of the concept of masochism—with a nod to influence of the pragmatist William James. The title links the idea of masochism to "experience" and "relating." I will not discuss the "masochistic personality" as a unitary disorder but rather as the kind of experiences such patients present to the analyst in the consultation room. I will not attempt here to give justice to the complexity and the historical evolution of the idea of masochism. Like other concepts in analysis (narcissism/transference, etc.), the word is very saturated and the boundaries not easy to see. Rather, I would like to show how the concept of masochism arises in my work with patients, found in the often subtle interactions between us, located in the transference-countertransference field. My approach will be pragmatic: what notions of masochism have, for me, the greatest "cash value" in the clinical encounter. By "cash value," I mean the concepts which allow me to be receptive to unconscious communications and able to better tolerate and reflect on my countertransference reactions. I will point to ways of working that may help these patients by way of clinical illustrations.

Masochistic experiences are expressions of unconscious object relations. These object relations derive from all levels of mental life, from the most primitive to the most evolved and organized. There is a core idea of masochistic experience I find useful in organizing my thinking. The masochistic experience offers *some form of pleasure in suffering* and is sought *over and over again.* This pleasure ("terrible delights") varies—excitement of all sorts (sexual, aggressive, narcissistic), as well as relief from terror and anxiety—so that the various forms of pleasure contribute to the complexity of the experience and difficulty for the analyst to find the right level to understand and interpret.

There is another important quality to the masochistic experience: the feeling of being *trapped, imprisoned, subjugated.* This sense of imprisonment may be at the hands of a sadistic internal object, a sadistic part of the self, a merged self/object, and is externalized through enactments with the analyst. *Dependence on and surrender* to this persecutory object/part of the self is involved in the suffering. The combination of pleasure in the experience, with a feeling of being trapped, often gives the subject the sense of being involved in something addictive, impossible to give up.

There are clinical and theoretical ideas that I have found useful in thinking about this core masochistic experience. What I want to do now is sketch some of these interrelated ideas. I rely on the concept of the death drive (vs. the life instincts) as described by Hannah Segal, Betty Joseph and Michael Feldman. Andre Green has made very important contributions in this area, but for the moment I will leave them aside; I will discuss his ideas on this subject later. Segal (1993), Joseph (1959, 1982) and Feldman (2000) emphasize that the clinical manifestation of the death drive is a refusal to face feelings of guilt, envy, anxiety, and uncertainty in the depressive position which arises from separation and dependency on a whole object. Segal expresses the conflict this way: "One, to seek gratification for the needs: that is life promoting and leads to object seeking, love, and eventual object concern. The other is the drive to annihilate the need, the perceiving experiencing self, as well as anything that is perceived" (p. 55). The death drive, "to annihilate need," is a psychological, not a biological concept. This annihilation involves a turn toward omnipotent phantasy and action which deny the pain and anxiety of separateness and dependency. The phantasies and actions are destructive and anti-life; in fact, there is a hatred of life and human experience. Segal adds that pleasure is involved: "there is also the satisfaction of triumph of the death-dealing part over the wish to live . . . not only the sadistic pleasure of triumph over the defeated analyst but also the masochistic pleasure over that part of oneself that wishes to live and grow" (p. 59). In terms of countertransference experiences with masochistic patients, Segal observes feeling paralyzed with a sense of deadness, or feeling pessimistic, despairing and aggressive toward the patient.

Joseph develops these clinical ideas further in a series of papers dealing with patients whose relationship to life and human objects is tenuous at best. In an early paper, Joseph (1959) notes that mastering anxiety involved in dependence on a primary or part object is achieved by "a particular balance between destructiveness and love, and how the very nature of this balance in itself can lead to no progress" (p. 17). Life is "lived" in "a state of paralysis, of suspended animation" (p. 33). This balance is achieved in the analytic relationship by keeping the object "internally paralyzed." The analyst presents a potential threat to this balance: "Each time these carriers of the life instinct disturb the patients' peace a situation akin to a trauma arises, and they react in a way which seems aimed at restoring their quasi-inorganic state" (p. 32). For this reason the analyst must be kept in a weakened state in the patient's mind; the patient enacts situations in which the analyst is perceived as weak and paralyzed.

In the paper "Addiction to near-death," Joseph vividly describes the working of the death instinct in masochism in a patient for whom "there is a felt need to know and have the satisfaction of seeing oneself being destroyed," in which "seeing the self in this dilemma, unable to be helped, is an essential aspect" (p. 449). Joseph analyzes the masochistic excitement of self-annihilation, which "annihilates also the object." The analyst invariably is caught up in this masochistic excitement through projective identification:

> Some patients present "real" situations, but in such a way as silently and extremely convincingly to make the analyst feel quite hopeless and despairing. The patient appears to feel the same. I think we have here a type of projective identification in which despair is so effectively loaded into the analyst that he seems crushed by it and can see no way out. The analyst is then internalized in this form by the patient, who becomes caught up in this internal crushing and crushed situation, and paralyses and deep gratification ensue. (p. 452)

In addition to these countertransference difficulties, Joseph finds that the patient splits off and projects onto the analyst "the pull toward life and sanity" which might pressure the analyst to rescue and want to enliven the patient and which further intensifies the gratification, and at times, excitement for the patient in creating these futile exchanges.

It is important, as Joseph emphasizes, to discern when the patient is communicating in such a way to "create a masochistic situation" and when the patient is communicating a state of hopelessness that he "wants us to understand and to help him with" (p. 453). I will discuss these technical questions below.

Feldman (2000) adds to this picture by underscoring that this sense of destructiveness is exciting and involves feelings of triumph and omnipotent control over a weakened object and the real effect this can have on the analyst's state of mind and behavior.[1] Feldman's contribution is to show how the scene for the masochistic narrative is unconscious and involves an unconscious attempt (often successfully) to actualize these phantasies with the analyst. Feldman finds in the clinical examples in the literature, and in his own work, the desire of the patient to weaken, torture and impoverish the object or the relationship with associated feelings of excitement, gratification, triumph and sense of power. The consequence of this attack is "the deadly way in which meaning… and differences are attacked and any developmental processes retarded or undermined" (p. 64). One of Feldman's gifts is to demonstrate how this shows up in the session and what the analyst must contend with in order to gain a position where the stirred-up affects and phantasies can be tolerated and used interpretively. He does not underestimate the pressure on the analyst to act out these phantasies with the patient by retaliating, withdrawing in despair or resorting to manic reparative efforts. Any and all of the reactions will feed the patient's triumphant excitement that, indeed, the analyst has been weakened in some way.

Segal, Joseph, and Feldman agree that the ultimate therapeutic aim is achieved through interpretation *which is only possible if the countertransference feelings can be tolerated,* and the analyst comes to understand what is enacted unconsciously between patient and analyst. Feldman suggests that once the analyst understands these underlying phantasies and gains a capacity to tolerate the position the patient puts him in, then interpretation "may bring these destructive activities into the realm of thought and language, thereby diminishing their silent destructiveness, and partly liberating his objects from their grip" (p. 65). Segal describes how an interpretation that put her patient in touch with an "almost direct experience of her own wish for total annihilation . . . lessened the persecution and put her in touch with the psychic reality of her own drives" (p. 57). Segal goes on: "a confrontation with the death instinct, in *favorable circumstances,* mobilizes the life instinct as well" (italics added). At another point Segal reiterates: "The experience [through interpretation] of the real consequences of giving in to this death drive mobilized his life forces in opposition" (p. 57).

What Feldman and Joseph add to Segal's view (and we see this in Green, Herbert Rosenfeld and Paul Williams below) is the perversely self-protecting aspect to the way the subject leans on and makes use of the death drive in masochism. As Joseph remarked, the disruption of the self's dependence on death-related phantasies can be felt as a trauma. This is suggested in Feldman's work also, where masochism protects the patient from overwhelming anxiety in facing separateness and dependency on an object outside the self.

The second concept I make use of is the model of pathological organizations of the self as described by Herbert Rosenfeld (1971, 1988). Rosenfeld describes a *stable structure of the self-organization,* in which one part of the self—libidinal, attached, dependent—is dominated by another part of the self which is tyrannical, cold, and sadistic and upon which the libidinal part of the self is dependent. He describes the setting in vivid terms as a mafia situation: the gang or dominant/sadistic part of the self is the mafia which offers "protection" to the libidinal self in exchange for undying loyalty and submission (1971). The nature of this relationship is sadomasochistic and relies on a threat of violence toward the libidinal part of the self. As a result, the analyst meets with a patient who cannot rely on the analyst or whose efforts to connect with the analyst are often obstructed by some destructive or self-destructive force whenever contact or progress is made. So the analyst is often confronted with negative therapeutic reactions. I want to note that this structure, the pathological organization, is very stable, and its stability depends on the fact that the libidinal part of the self relies on the gang. This gang derives from different sources: as a primitive superego, as an intrusive object related to traumatic experience, as a merger with a powerful persecutory parental figure (or couple) or as a manic part of the self. It is important for the analyst to get what kind of object this is as the work proceeds. John Steiner (1982) and Rosenfeld point out that the dependent part of the self participates in the relationship in a masochistic and perverse way to maintain the status quo. Rosenfeld (1988) states: "there must be reasons and tendencies in those parts of the self that submit to the domination and imprisonment" (p. 151). He goes on:

> A sadomasochistic situation is created where the infantile self of the patient is left to painful suffering, starvation and poisoning. The attacks on the infantile part of the self and its suffering are obviously increased to triumph over the important objects that have to watch the infant suffer without being able to help and save him from death. (p. 152)

This sadomasochistic situation is recreated with the analyst: there is withdrawal from real objects and an addiction to powerful destructive self-states. The analyst represents a threat because "Contact with me meant a weakening of narcissistic omnipotent superiority . . . which was avoided by detachment" (p. 153).

Rosenfeld emphasizes: "these patients, who should be regarded as potentially psychotic, are not aware that the pull into the psychotic state implies a pull toward death" (p. 154). This psychotic state however excited or active, is detached from real objects; the subject is completely absorbed by an inner sadomasochistic drama with which the analyst is not meant to interfere. Moments of contact with the analyst are followed by a "psychotic, destructive narcissistic structure or self that threatened her whenever she attempted to come closer to life or any living person" (p. 155). Rosenfeld is describing a perverse inhuman inner world that prevents the subject from relating to live human objects. One perverse aspect is the way the psychotic structure of the self propagandizes and creates panic whenever real relating is immanent.

Paul Williams (2010) has provided a rich understanding as to why this pathological organization persists and why its disruption is felt as traumatic. In conditions of incorporation of an invasive object (which is terrifying and persecuting and may be related to the "gang"), separation represents a potential loss of the "ongoing sense of self" and so feels catastrophic. As trauma figures importantly in William's contributions, the suggestion is that the basic survival of the self involves a merger with an object/structure, a pathological organization, to protect the self from traumatic experiences of intrusion or abandonment. "Genuine sustained dialogue" represents a threat to what is felt essential to the patient. He emphasizes the need for the analyst to tolerate prolonged periods of uncertainty and confusion, as contact is rare with masochistically withdrawn patients.

The third concept, which is foundational to the idea of a pathological organization, is one developed by W. R. Bion. Bion (1957) describes a kind of heterogeneous self in which there resides a psychotic and a non-psychotic part of the personality. The psychotic part of the personality hates reality and development, destroys the capacity to think (and thus appreciate reality) in herself—and in the analyst at times—while there continues to survive a sane part of the personality striving to think and know the truth. These parts of the personality are not integrated. The level of integration determines a lot of what the clinical encounter looks like.

These ideas suggest a motivation behind masochistic experience, a turning away from the contingencies of life, away from pain, loss, mourning, separateness, and the responsibility which comes with loving. From the patient's point of view, these withdrawn self-destructive states are felt as necessary, and the experience of anything else is foreign and threatening.

There is one final note here regarding a phenomenon that looks masochistic but primarily involves narcissistic structures. Green (1999), in his description of the death drive, shows how overt masochism conceals a profound narcissistic withdrawal. This narcissistic withdrawal is in fact the death drive: a decathexis, a "disobjectalizing function" in which the subject is suffering, but there is no object, only a movement toward non-existence. This distinction is important, and I hope to illustrate its significance with clinical material.

In my view, where we find this masochistic experience and way of relating, which can often be very subtle, is in what is being lived out with the analyst, and particularly, what is happening at each moment in the session. As a generalization of the course of the work with masochistic patients, there is a movement from a lived-out sadomasochistic relationship with the analyst to one in which the patient acknowledges they are relying on something destructive within him or herself which eventually is felt as distressing and frightening, to seeking the analyst's help. Of course, that movement can happen over years or minutes, and it is not linear. The analyst's attention is paid in each session to the movement of these states and internal relationships, from excited triumph to anxiety about the nature of their destructiveness, to a more realistic mode of relating to the analyst. The analyst often has the sense the patient is relying on something internally (or externally acted out) that has the quality of an addiction which the person feels powerless to give up (and does not know it).

It is only by carefully analyzing this structure that is lived out with the analyst—which is often perverse—that we may eventually find out about the nature of the underlying anxieties, lack of self-cohesion, unconscious phantasies and possible traumatic experiences. I view the subject seeking masochistic experiences as a solution, and what the masochistic world is trying to solve can only be glimpsed once the patient has reached the point of separating somewhat from it. I am making this much more schematic than it actually is in the consultation room, of course, where there is a mixture of experience, and often, confusion.

A final note: part of the masochistic solution requires that the patient's object remain either powerless, "kept in an internally paralyzed state" to quote Joseph, muted or deadened or impotently sadistic. That is, the analyst is often enticed to feel and act in ways (unconsciously) which strengthen the pathological organization. An essential of the work for the analyst is in grasping this aspect of the countertransference, tolerating and reflecting, so as to disrupt the equilibrium. On the other hand, what brings the patient for analysis ultimately is a sane part of him that is trapped in something he is powerless to change, which should be at least silently acknowledged by the analyst.

CLINICAL EXAMPLES

Dr. N is a married man in his early thirties who came for treatment because he felt burdened by life and could take no pleasure in it. He seemed to be liked by colleagues, patients, and friends, as well as by his wife, but had little interest in deepening these relationships. He sought time alone, "to be left alone," for his solitary projects, and yet when he had time, he often was unable to make use of the time in a productive way. He described being paralyzed with obsessional doubt during his free time. He relayed images of his life in a vague, two-dimensional way. I could never grasp what it was really like, but the tone was usually grim and barren. In short, he seemed masochistic in that any of life's pleasures immediately turned painful.

The story of his family and childhood had the same vagueness and grimness. Both parents were busy, successful professionals but seemed to have very little expectation for or interest in Dr. N, the oldest of three siblings. His narrative was unwavering and rote each time as he told me how his father was too busy to help him with his work or his mother too narcissistically involved in her social life. It is not that these pictures seemed irrelevant to me, but rather that they were lifeless, static depictions which never changed. The narrative was meant to account for why Dr. N felt so little passion. He did convey a sense of deadness in his inner world, and his objects seemed empty and lifeless. Though I knew this could not be the whole story, either of his life outside analysis, his childhood, or his inner world, in the consultation room an oppressive sense of futility and lifelessness pervaded the atmosphere.

The analysis began with Dr. N conveying a thin idealization of me in which he felt small and lacking in all ways in comparison to me—sexually, intellectually, creatively. If I attempted to point out this idealization which led to his sense of inferiority, Dr. N was adamant in the reality of his perception of himself and me. He would account for this by citing his impoverished emotional background and assuming I had loving, indulgent parents who fostered my development. I was meant to accept these descriptions without question.

Gradually, over time, we settled into something negative and static. Dr. N, as a result of my attempts to open up the meaning of his narratives, felt that I did not understand him, in part because we came from two different worlds: I from the haves and Dr. N from the have-nots. Whenever I could show him how motivated his view of each of us was—to escape a sense of anxiety with me, to rid himself of anything positive, etc.—it seemed to intensify his need to insist that I could not understand him and his lack, that I could not understand it because I did not feel the sort of lack someone like Dr. N would feel. Though if I accepted his sense of lack, he would rail against me for my complacency.

In this part of the work my words were meant to reach him and end his suffering or at least enlighten us to the reasons for it. Dr. N had an almost uncanny sense of when I felt attached to what I said, and it was especially at those moments that he would convey a deeper sense of futility in our work. If I commented on the way he made use of what I said, or perhaps why (to defeat me, impoverish me, etc.) by draining it of life, he would violently reject those comments: "I can't do that to you. You are the powerful one here, not me. You have it all together—I'm the schmo. . . . [W]ho'd want to help a schmo." This way of relating undermined any understanding between us, protecting him from change while also allowing him to feel powerful in his weakness. By effortlessly expressing his envy of me, having a more real sense of his emotions was impossible at this time. A seamless impenetrability met my efforts to make contact.

What is important to capture here is that the emotional climate was altogether different from the words spoken between us. Although he strenuously argued that his experience left him irremediably empty, lacking and hopeless and that I had so much, my feelings were at odds with this. I felt quite frustrated and constrained with him. I had few ideas and fantasies in his presence that seemed alive. I was struggling to find some way of understanding and reaching him, and my efforts were feeling more and more futile. Dr. N, on the other hand, seemed comfortable, if not relaxed, and articulated the paradox that *I was lacking in understanding of his inferiority.* This involved a subtle provocation: the more I cared about helping him and feeling I had something to offer him, the more despairing (and disparaging) he became. He would relate how his life was only getting worse, that he was feeling more dead and hopeless, that he was giving up on activities that once offered some minimal form of pleasure. Perhaps, he mused, psychoanalysis is a sham, a Ponzi scheme to extract money from helpless folks like him. Things like this were said frequently but not in a paranoid way. The quality was more that now, he is in the know, onto the way really things are, onto me, and is in fact feeling superior. I felt ensnared by his way of relating: suffering, helpless, in constant pain but with this glimmer of superiority. I had difficulty finding an emotional place of freedom. And the verbal messages from him were contradictory and sparse: no dreams, no accounts of vital outside activities or relationships, no vivid memories. All the action was in the emotional climate we shared. As Bion (1979) states: "When two personalities meet, an emotional storm is created." This storm was quiet yet devastating. It then gathered steam.

Dr. N began a campaign to show the way that I was, in his words, "an empty suit." Through the Internet he found out as much as he could about me. He used this information to show that, despite my reputation and apparent confidence, I was probably useless and could not help him, even though I *seemed* content and successful. What was subtle before became obviously envious and hateful. He would find information on the Internet about me, things which I felt quite good or even proud of—a paper, bar mitzvah, etc.—and be able to spoil any positive feelings I had about it. At this he was a master, all the while acting as if I merited being the object of his envy. I find it hard, except through the concept of projective identification, to conceptualize the powerful, negative impact he had on my mood. Areas in which I would naturally feel good or at least satisfied became a source of shame and hopelessness. This was, of course, a glimpse of his internal world and persecutory objects, but I could only emotionally maintain that view in a consistent way outside the sessions.

Beyond the feeling of hopelessness he engendered in me, I also felt a real sense of persecution. His Internet researches evoked a hyper self-consciousness that many of my activities were within his destructive reach. My interpretations became confrontational and sharp. The content of these interpretations was accurate yet motivated by a defensive desire to push him back. These interpretations fueled his excitement and also apparent despair: "I know I'm being destructive and bad. But why can't you help me stop this. You're the expert here. It's not like I want to be this way! That's why I'm here for help." At these moments, his moods rapidly shifted from anger to hopelessness. And I had the sense that nothing I could say would do anything but further an endless series of point-counterpoint comments. If on occasion I had managed to capture something in him that disrupted for a moment this masochistic structure, he would pause, look touched, and then utter: "Why didn't you say that before? This must have been obvious to you for some time. Were you withholding that?"

When I examined what was going on outside the sessions, I could momentarily gain a perspective of what he was communicating to me of his internal world: the concepts of projective identification and pathological organizations helped me understand the grandiose, persecutory, devaluing internal object which stripped the subject/patient of any sense of worth, internal goodness, or sense of liveliness. This persecutory object/organization hated his desire for contact with me and growth. Yet in the session, the intensity of the transference-countertransference field limited my ability to reflect on my experience and contain it. As a result of this difficulty, I think we enacted in subtle ways a sadomasochistic object relationship which was stabilizing to him.

Increasingly, I began to sense *in the session* the threat and potential terror I posed to him and the masochistic structure which protected him. This happened as a result of tolerating the feelings of persecution and hopelessness. I gradually felt calmer. I think what was very important in this transition was the feeling that I did not need to save him, that my interpretations did not need to *do* anything.

I felt less compelled to offer something useful to him, to prove my utility and goodness, to intuit a transformative interpretation. Bion (1994) states that interpretations should come from a sense of feeling content, and I was able to feel a sense of contentment in tolerating what I felt and thought about it without doing anything.

As my perspective changed, I could see and calmly comment on the patient's excitement in expressing his suffering to me. The most important factor is not the content or observations I made, but the state of mind I conveyed to him in my comments. That is, I communicated a sense of tolerance and acceptance of his inner world. What was tolerated was a persecutory, deadening object that I think he contended with all the time. As long as I defended against that aspect of himself, I could not really help him with it. I also conveyed (more in attitude than words) how much he relied on this omnipotent way of suffering. His manic suffering increased initially in response to my changing state of mind, as he sensed that I was no longer paralyzed by the atmosphere between us. I could better tolerate the excited, defensive states he brought to me, to keep me at a distance, and so could make calm and somewhat detached observations.

Here is a fragment from a session during this period of transition, from enactment to containment: "This weekend was horrible as usual. I couldn't do anything. I wanted to paint but couldn't get myself to do it. You don't see how badly off I am. I can't really paint. I can't. You have a ridiculous dream that I can, that it might work, that it is worthwhile, but that is ridiculous." (He is getting more energetic and excited as he describes himself in this hapless way. Really, we are a hapless pair together). I point out this excitement—that it makes him excited to describe this weakness to me, to be weak with me. As I begin to pick up on this and firmly and calmly point it out, he becomes irritable and then, very gradually, I can detect a sense of relief.

We went through this cycle many times, which I described to him in a somewhat neutral way: his excitement in expressing his/my weakness and lack, his resistance to my observation, then a growing sense of calm or at least a more relaxed state as I am not put off by his reactions. I think my taking a strong stand on what I observed was a communication that an object that can stand up to the destructiveness without negotiation but in a calm, receptive, and non-retaliatory way. I did not interpret the underlying motivation, which I had done in the past. Aside from conveying my frustration or defensiveness at times, those sorts of interpretations were also meant to get him to see and stop what he was doing, which fed his sense of excitement and power.

In a schematic way, I will describe a transition from the hold the pathological organization had on Dr. N to a way of relating to me as a separate helpful object. Dr. N's excitement evolved into anxiety. He became concerned that his destructiveness could demolish any good feeling inside him. He noticed how his desires or needs were especially targeted—ridiculed and mocked. He began to feel protective of good experiences or feelings, and for the first time, he could tell me something good about himself or his life, as he also acknowledged his fragile hold on it: "You will remember this for me, because I can't." At this point in the analysis, he turned to me for real help. What was an external battle between us—or rather a stable structure of two weakened merged objects dominated by a sadistic force—became an internal one.

What emerged, what he could then describe, was a vicious, devaluing part of him that drained the life out of any impulse or desire to the point where that alive part of the self felt useless and dying. He experienced this destructive part of himself as very powerful and exciting. For example, he described a certain kind of excitement in watching the two of us "flail" and make no progress. There was an internal sense of victory and triumph over anything alive, tender, or hopeful. The more he could describe this aspect of his experience, the more distance he gained (in parallel to what I had gone through). He said: "There are three of us here, and one always watches, demeans, ridicules, mocks."

This part of the treatment was very alive and volatile, and I could see the moment-to-moment shifts in his self-states depending on his relation to the destructive part of him and his relationship to me. Because he had weakened me in phantasy, he was unsure whether I was strong enough to help him and stand up to this destructiveness. I could track the vicissitudes of this sense of his analyst at each moment. It was very important to determine whether his concern for me represented something genuine and a real anxiety or the destructive/psychotic part of him relishing in my weakness.

Even though we could predict a backlash to progress when he was captured or in thrall to this destructive part of him, he had no access at that moment to anything else, as if he had fallen into another world. I observed with him the way he might exaggerate a disappointment, or propagandize against me and the analysis.

As Rosenfeld (1988) observed, contact with the analyst means weakening of "narcissistic omnipotent superiority." Rosenfeld also describes with great accuracy that the patient initially does not know about this destructive part, how enticing or psychotic it is because "it is posed as a friend." The self can find strength and protection from an identification and/or merger with an intrusive object, an identification or merger that in the past was felt as the sole means of surviving. Separation from this powerful, omnipotent object is met with terror. We had to work again, each time, at reinstating a connection to me and, each time, re-experienced his anxiety at the power of his destructiveness. Often, it felt as if he had awakened from a partially dissociated state.

Once Dr. N could tolerate the anxiety engendered by contact with me, we could explore the nature and function of his phantasies as they emerged in the transference communications and dreams. The content of his phantasies involved grandiose, triumphant victory over weakened parental figures. Often, he was identified with the maternal figure. The function of these phantasies protected him from relating to and caring for real objects he could not control or he might lose. Disruption of the masochistic experience exposed him to the terrifying risk of caring for someone else he could not control or could lose. We could not analyze in an emotionally connected way these phantasies until he had gained a certain level of freedom from his masochistic world.

In the termination phase, which lasted about a year and a half, Dr. N gained a tolerance for feelings and recognition of the grandiose nature of his phantasies. He could begin to express real love and concern for the people in his life.

I would like to contrast Dr. N with a patient who is in the grip of the death drive, but in a more narcissistic way, as Andre Green (1999) describes. In this case, my interventions were different, but eventually led to the kind of work I described with Dr. N.

E is a twenty-year-old female student who came to analysis with symptoms of deadness and depersonalization. As she gradually attached to me, the separations became unbearable. Before analysis, E had unconsciously resolved to decathect from all objects and activities, going through life in a zombie-like state. She smoked copious amounts of marijuana to sustain her deadness. As she started to come alive in the analysis, we could see the vicissitudes of the death drive. What I mean is that moments of separation in the session (psychically) or between sessions led to feelings of emptiness—an objectless state she described as a dark hole without life or light. It was important for me to understand that at these moments she was not "taken over" or "subjugated" but rather alone and fragmented. This kind of state requires a more alive, active presence from the analyst.

As she emerged from this narcissistic state in the course of the analysis, as she came more alive and could sense me as a real person, a masochistic experience took its place to protect her from these objectless states: a merged state with a tyrannical maternal figure she relied on when separated from me. Her actual mother had been sick most of her life, often remaining in bed for days in a darkened room. E would lie close to her in silence, and it was when her mother was most "out of it" with her illness that she could tolerate the closeness with her daughter. At other times, the mother was described as volatile and brittle, critical and rejecting. So during any sort of break in time, empathy, or lack of complete access to me, she turned to the suffering state—deadness and quiet merger. To die is to live with mother. This intrusive object hated anything alive in E.

The analysis then took the turn similar to Dr. N: an analysis of a pathological organization, though in E's case, a personality much less integrated where the psychotic experience was more pervasive, so the enactments between us were less formed and my countertransference feelings more chaotic, extreme, and unformed. For E, it was preferable to rely on/merge with a powerful deadening maternal figure than rely on a real person who could leave, misunderstand, etc. When she merged with this psychotic part of her personality, there was *great relief in seeing all that she relied on in me and in her reduced to ashes, a relief that also gave her a feeling of triumph and superiority.* I could not interpret this sense of relief because her experience was more like she had been taken over and could not think or articulate what was going on. She would often come into sessions as if living in another world, and we were strangers to each other. She had no memory of past experiences and no desire for anything. Though for E this masochistic experience protected her from an objectless terrifying world, the masochistic state was much more fragmented and psychotic than the world that Dr. N's masochistic relating offered. Her masochistic experience encased her. In those moments, there was no one to talk to. In phantasy, the analyst was put into the position of a helpless witness, which intensified her merged state and added a sense of power.

But as we began to make more contact and she felt moments of aliveness in the session—this occurred over a couple of years—a different form of masochistic experience emerged. She seemed more differentiated from her object world. Rather than a merged experience that encased and deadened her, she reacted to the analytic work and our relationship as a real threat and a more differentiated persecutory object emerged, more like the object—the "gang"—that Rosenfeld described. This internal object ridiculed anything she desired and left her feeling humiliated. At first, her relationship to this object was perverse excitement. The result of this process though was for her to feel in great conflict between her need for contact with me that left her more alive and hopeful and her attraction to states of abject misery and mortification, at which time our work and her desires for life were experienced as laughable. The work then was to notice the sense of power that her inner, perverse world offered her, that made "real life" seem paltry. The perverse aspect to this relating felt euphoric in that reality could be turned upside down, where suffering and failure were virtues, where real life experiences were made unreal. This went for the analytic relationship as well. At any moment, E could feel as if we were enacting some play that had no meaning for her. She had a dream in which during an analytic session she noticed a cameraman in the corner of the office filming us. The man had a beard, which she associated to Coppola filming Martin Sheen, in the film *Apocalypse Now*. The association to the film carried the sense of a sane part of her that knew that this "unreality" was the work of a part of her called "Apocalypse Now." This dream suggested an initial separation from the part of her intoxicated with destruction and the manipulation of reality.

As with Dr. N, when I could show her the pleasure in the power to reduce anything of value to nothing, the sane part of her became much more anxious and sought my help. She began to hate that part of herself she identified with her mother and very gradually gained distance from it.

CONCLUSION

I would like to summarize the main points in this paper:

1. Masochistic experience is finding pleasure in suffering at the hands of a powerful, destructive internal object, in which the experience of being trapped or imprisoned is central.
2. The dependence on this masochistic experience, which is often addictive, protects against differing sorts of anxieties and self-states which can only be fully recognized and analyzed once the masochistic experience is disrupted.
3. The analyst inevitably and often unknowingly participates in the masochistic experience, which strengthens its hold.
4. The self and the "gang," psychotic part or a destructive internal object have different qualities and account for the range of masochistic phenomena in our work.
5. The psychotic part propagandizes/dominates/imprisons the sane non-psychotic part. The sane part can relate in different ways to this destructive part that is more or less differentiated from a rapport to a merged state.
6. In this way, there are differing levels and manifestations of masochism due to differing levels of integration.

NOTE

1. Feldman's view of the way the analyst is inevitably taken up by the patient's influence is more fully described in his "Projective Identification: The Analyst's Involvement (1997).

REFERENCES

Bion, W. R. (1957). Differentiation of the psychotic from the non-psychotic personalities. *International Journal of Psychoanalysis* 38: 266–75.

—— (1959). Attacks on linking. *International Journal of Psychoanalysis* 40: 308–15.

—— (1979). Making the best of a bad job. In *Clinical Seminars and Other Works*. London: Karnac Books, 2000.

—— (1994). *Clinical Seminars and Other Works*. London: Karnac Books

—— (1997). Projective identification: The analyst's involvement. *International Journal of Psycho-Analysis* 78: 227–41

—— (2000). Some views on the manifestation of the death instinct in clinical work. *International Journal of Psychoanalysis* 81: 53–65.

Feldman, M. (1994). Projective identification in phantasy and enactment. *Psychoanalytic Inquiry* 14: 423–40.

—— (2000). Some views on the manifestation of the death instinct in clinical work. *International Journal of Psychoanalysis* 81: 53–65.

Freud, S. (1916). On transience. *Standard Edition* 14: 303–7.

—— (1917). Mourning and melancholia. *Standard Edition* 14: 237–58.

—— (1919). A child is being beaten. *Standard Edition* 18: 175–204.

—— (1920). Beyond the pleasure principle. *Standard Edition* 18: 1–64.

—— (1924). The economic problem of masochism. *Standard Edition* 19: 155–70.

Green, A. (1999). The death drive, negative narcisissm, and the disobjectalizing function. In *The Work of the Negative*. London: Free Association Books.

Joseph, B. (1959). An aspect of the repetition compulsion. *International Journal of Psychoanalysis* 40: 1–10.

—— (1982). Addiction to near-death. *International Journal of Psychoanalysis* 63: 449–56.

Rosenfeld, H. (1971). A clinical approach to the psychoanalytic theory of the life and death instincts: An investigation into the aggressive aspects of narcissism. *International Journal of Psychoanalysis* 52: 169–78.

—— (1988). On masochism: A theoretical and clinical approach. In *Masochism: Current Psychoanalytic Perspectives*, eds. R. Glick and D. Meyers, D. Hillsdale, NJ: Analytic Press.

Segal, H. (1993). On the clinical usefulness of the concept of the death instinct. *International Journal of Psychoanalysis* 74: 55–61.

Steiner, J. (1982). Perverse relationships between parts of the self: A clinical illustration. *International Journal of Psychoanalysis* 63: 241–51.

Williams, P. (2010). *Invasive Objects: Minds Under Siege*. London: Routledge.

NINE

Masochism and Trauma

Harold P. Blum, MD

This paper will explore masochistic fantasy underlying masochistic phenomena as influenced by severe, protracted trauma. The traumatic experience has usually begun in early life, with additive traumas in subsequent developmental phases. Masochism is a compromise formation encompassing numerous determinants and factors. Conscious masochistic fantasy—for instance, a beating fantasy or a fantasy of bondage or self-injury—represents a complex of conflicts, developmental disturbances, adaptive and mal-adaptive maneuvers. Trauma figures prominently in the development of masochism and sadism in many cases but is not a unitary or unifying explanation. Aspects of masochism continue to be mysterious, awaiting further illumination from multi-disciplinary research. For purposes of this paper, masochism is defined as consciously or unconsciously seeking pain, suffering, and humiliation. Most symptoms are unpleasant and distressing, without masochism necessarily being most important in the underlying conflicts. Masochism and sadism are always paired in the psyche, and this coalescence is exemplified in the concept of "sadomasochism."

The wide variety of masochistic manifestations—for example, head-banging, self-cutting, self-defeating behaviors, familial and marital battles, severely restricted gratifications, etc.—attests to its many determinants, meanings, and functions (Brenner, 1959), (Maleson, 1984). The partnership of masochism, sadism, and narcissism is relatively universal; they can alternate and defend against each other. They are present in degree in all persons, frequently represented by a conscious or unconscious beating fantasy. The pleasure found in the wide depiction of violence in the media, as well as the high incidence of domestic violence and cruelty, is indicative of the pervasive sadomasochism of everyday life (Ross, 1997). Though not elaborated in clinical theory and discourse, there are important cultural and social dimensions to masochism, so evident in institutionalized slavery, racism, and the subjugation of nations in colonialism. Sadomasochism has been closely associated with the power gradients of social class and the humiliation of disparaged, devalued minorities at the intersection of cultural stereotype and personal identity (Kucich, 2006). Extreme forms of sadomasochistic cruelty, dehumanization and demonization were apparent in the Holocaust and in all too many other man-made disasters.

I shall focus here on clinical examples and theoretical exposition in which masochism is predominant, interrelated to psychic and physical trauma (Glenn, 1984). Regarding sadomasochism, it certainly makes a difference in terms of external and internal conflict whether a person seeks personal pain and suffering, seeks affection and sympathy or primarily tries to inflict pain and suffering on others. Social and legal consequences are far more commonly concomitants of sadistic behaviors.

For purposes of this paper, trauma is defined as a state in which the ego is overwhelmed and reduced to relative helplessness and loss of function. Severe shock trauma or protracted stress trauma may result in concurrent physical as well as psychological collapse or impairment may be relative with different effects on various ego functions. Trauma may be acute, recurrent or persistent with ensuing cumulative trauma. Cumulative trauma may be punctuated by episodes of shock and strain trauma. In the cases to be described, severe, massive trauma extending in time through different developmental phases, periods of life, and relationships was recurrent and cumulative. Pathogenic object relations may be the most common form of masochistic expression, representing and contributing to sadomasochistic conflicts and to the development of masochistic character and personality disorders.

CASE I: MASOCHISM IN ANOREXIA NERVOSA

The pathogenesis of anorexia nervosa has been the subject of long-standing analytic and medical investigations, and I shall not attempt to review the literature and explanatory theories. See Zerbe (1993) for a thorough explication of psychoanalytic approaches to the treatment of the condition. Anorexia nervosa, or self-starvation, is an eating disorder with prominent self-destructive features though little discussed in terms of masochism. I will highlight the early infantile and childhood sadomasochistic-traumatic experience which was a major component of the subsequent adolescent anorexia. Most individuals who have been starved because of illness or famine do not repeat the trauma through self-starvation. Furthermore, formerly anorexic patients are not usually inclined to starve others, or to reverse the trauma and force feed other persons or pets or to encourage obesity. Combined bulimia/anorexia may be a variant condition with a related pathogenesis but not necessarily entailing starvation. What I especially want to emphasize in this and related cases of severe masochistic anorexia is the painful primary object relationship. This anorexic patient was the daughter of upper-middle-class parents who were well educated and consciously devoted to their daughter's welfare and what they considered to be proper child-rearing practices. The mother reported a normal pregnancy and delivery, without any major problems of nausea, weight gain or medical complication. Length of pregnancy and birth weight were normal, and the baby was briefly breast-fed followed by an unremarkable transfer to a bottle. The baby was placid, but alert, with a very brief and mild form of colic. Her mother did not favor demand feeding, and a reportedly brief amount of fussing and crying was permitted, especially if the last feeding was "recent." This pattern of non-intervention to alleviate the infant's distress and crying was continued and intensified during the patient's toddler period. Her mother had strict rules concerning discipline. Even minor infractions could result in the girl's being sent to her room. Her mother experienced little pleasure in body contact or holding her infant, and felt little distress in her infant's distress. While "proper" discipline might have seemed harsh to others, including the girl's father, the mother was not dissuaded from her dutiful promotion of discipline and her militant rigidity. As a result, the little girl was subject to separation and isolation in the prison of her bedroom. She would then cry incessantly until she fell asleep exhausted. The next day her mother would be affectionate, sometimes playful, as though nothing had happened. All of her fruitless and helpless cries seemed to be forgotten by mother and daughter. Her mother was not aware of guilt or remorse but rather prideful of preserving discipline and teaching her daughter respectful obedience. Significantly, persistent screaming and enraged crying in the infancy of patients with anorexia occurs with a relatively high frequency (Brody, 2001). That anorexia nervosa is far more common in females than males may be related to hostile, mother-daughter bonding, cultural inhibition of female external aggression and cultural emphasis on the female body and thin figure.

Toilet training and lessons in impulse and affect control were quickly successful in her second year; by age six or seven the patient was a model of relative independence, correct behavior and a superior student. In school her conduct was exemplary; she was the "teacher's pet," as she was mother's helper, a "goody two-shoes." On rare occasions when she opposed her mother, for example, regarding television time or overextended frivolous games, she would be reprimanded or even sent to her room with an abbreviated supper. Actually, she already had perfectionistic tendencies noted in many anorexics. She picked at her cuticles but did not have a history of thumb-sucking, nail-biting or an infant eating disorder; but her speech, mannerisms and gestures were careful and cautious. She lacked spontaneity and playful interactions; she was too serious with highly restricted, bland affect and facial expressions, more given to frowns than smiles.

Although the patient did not have an eating disorder as an infant, by latency idiosyncratic eating habits had appeared. Seemingly uncaring about her meals and denying her preoccupation with eating, she was picky and rigid in her choice of foods. While she denied her preoccupation with eating, consistent with many reports of anorexics, she ate slowly, chewing her food and keeping it in her mouth at length. Her excessive chewing and delayed swallowing actually increased her mealtime. Her actual preoccupation with food in certain respects echoed attitudes of her mother. The latter was a collector of cookbooks, decorated plates and recipes from foreign cultures. She had cultivated "taste," carefully choosing her recipes and restaurants. She thought her daughter would emulate her in culinary discrimination.

The patient's mother seemed oblivious to her daughter's stilted compliance and excessive need for her mother's approval, affection and engulfing attention. The patient's fragile self-esteem and her lack of self-confidence and self-reliance were not apparent to her family. However, some of her friends were aware of her fragility behind her external composure and her tearful responses to minor disappointments. Her father tried to be supportive and encouraging but left his daughter's childrearing mainly in the hands of the "devoted" mother. He thus failed to compensate for his wife's rigidity, nor did he sufficiently protect his daughter from her mother's insensitive discipline. As a consequence, the ambivalent enmeshment with her mother was intensified, setting the stage for her adolescent decompensation. Her bisexual identification with her father was pale in comparison to her primary, massive identification with her mother.

When this patient reached puberty at about twelve years of age, she was frightened by the visible changes in her body and the mysterious, surprising onset of menarche. Her mother had left preparation and discussion of menarche to the school nurse and school movies. What she heard from older girls engendered feelings of anxiety and humiliation. She knew she could eventually become pregnant, but this thought was equally as distressing as it was pleasurably exciting. She became petulant, fretful, and overly concerned with her figure and food. Noticeably different from the patient, her female classmates began to use cosmetics and were proud of their budding breasts and boys' attention to their changing bodies. Her parents at first hardly noticed that their daughter was becoming thin beyond the cultural ideal of the feminine figure. Her weight loss was very gradual and seemingly without any conscious awareness or concern. By the time she was approaching fourteen years of age her anorexia had become apparent. She was by then too thin for comfort and her menstrual periods had become short, scant, and irregular. Her parents finally became concerned, and her mother had her examined by the pediatrician who diagnosed anorexia nervosa. Her condition did not yield to medication, entreaties, bribes, or insistent commands to eat. She claimed to be indifferent to food and without appetite. She had gradually become dangerously underweight and anemic.

P began psychoanalytic psychotherapy and slowly began to gain weight concurrent with her analytic psychotherapy. Her long-apparent need to be perfect also meant being mistress of her passions, entailing repression of her hatred of herself and her parents. Treatment soon revealed that beneath her masochistic self-sacrifice lay her disowned and repressed insatiable hunger, not for food, but for love. Her internalized aggression toward her mother, and her mother's hostility toward her, became evident both within and outside the transference (Berliner 1958). She wanted to remain a sweet, dependent girl, an innocent victim of fate. She swallowed her anger but not her food. Direct, overt anger at her mother was internalized, but her rejection of food was a disguised, angry rejection of her mother. Similarly, she would not be overtly angry with her therapist but reject his feeding of clarification and interpretation. Her mother's rigidity and insensitivity—that is, not noticing her daughter's dangerous weight loss—had components of anger and hostility toward her daughter. Becoming a woman meant separation-individuation from her mother and competing with her mother for the love of her father. While feeling mildly distressed about her sickly state, she denied and minimized her suffering. She was inwardly gratified to remain physically and mentally a child. Her internal anguish periodically emerged. She felt like crying and screaming for no apparent reason and at times became tearful. She could not relate these bouts of crying to her current life or childhood. She knew "in her gut" that the depth of her distress could not be simply explained as seeking to arouse the therapist's and mother's guilt and pity. Her body was a messenger, and she was limited in being able to express affect verbally; she defended against affect recognition and expression through isolation and reaction formation. P attempted magical control of herself and her object world (Novick and Novick. 1996). In narcissistic fantasy she magically restored self-esteem and triumphed over a hostile, competitive, controlling maternal representation. The perfect, compliant self was split off from the hateful, rageful self, and the idealized mother was dissociated from the bad, hateful, maternal representation.

As the analytic psychotherapy proceeded, P began to experience her attenuated anguish and pain with less sugar coating, denial and dissociation. She was able to very gradually confront the perfectionism with which she attempted to compensate for impaired self-esteem and self-injury. Her masochistic/narcissistic character (Cooper. 1988) had paradoxical components of subjugated defeat and omnipotent victory.

Though her more mature self wanted to be helped to gain weight and insight, she also wanted to remain infantile. At times she was concerned, but at other times appeared indifferent to her condition. A secondary gain of the anorexia was to gain parental attention and psychiatric care and to punish her parents. Her rejection of food was a rejection of the "bad mother" figure and a silent assertion of a body ego independent of her mother. At the same time, she desperately wanted the "good mother" figure's love and approval. She belittled her own achievements which might lead into adolescent progression and revived oedipal rivalry. She was on a "mission impossible" between masochistic self-sacrifice and developmental advance. She wanted to be self-sustaining while self-starved; not hungry while internally greedy and devouring. P hurt herself through her self-starvation; starved for love, she also starved her internalized objects. P's later fantasies of oral impregnation through sucking and swallowing her father's milk/semen had a screening function. The fellatio fantasy defended against awareness of her oral fixation to the maternal object. These adolescent fantasies were initially unconscious and emerged from analysis of her dreams, daydreams, and her interest in popsicles and poppy seeds. On a pre-oedipal level, pregnancy would magically restore mother-infant union, as well as a wished-for and dreaded permanent childhood

The patient's experience of the therapist as a radically different new object, listening and responding with empathy and comprehension, were likely to have been beneficial determinants of her recovery alongside the dynamic, deeper analytic effects of clarification, interpretation, and insight. How much change in the masochistic personality structure occurred, and whether the infant and childhood stress trauma had enduring psychological and neurobiological sequela, remain open questions. Given present views of the resilience and the plasticity of the brain, many impairments of function may be relatively reversible due to treatment and subsequent favorable life experience. Some extremely traumatized children prove to be surprisingly resilient, and some borderline children develop into more highly functioning adults. Did the patient's endowment coalesce with the negative parental characteristics contributing to her symptoms and masochistic character? Was the anorexia nervosa related to a false self (Winnicott, 1965) and to an underlying depression? Her bland affect with regard to her anorexia appeared to defend against painful emotions of anxiety, rage, and depression (Blos, 1991; Blum, 1991). With more questions than answers, I believe that cumulative trauma was a critical determinant of P's masochistic character and her symptomatic anorexia nervosa. Early cumulative trauma contributes to the preponderance of aggression with fear of one's own aggression and possible retaliation (Parens, 1979). Sadomasochism is promoted and amplified. P's mother's love was contingent on her daughter's conformity; non-compliance was a threat to her mother, promoting aggression and punishment. Internalization and somatization of anger, as well as the maternal lack of apology, empathy or regret, all contributed to the girl's masochistic disposition. Her mother's angry withdrawal of love fortified the masochism and impeded the mastery of aggression. The inhibition of recreation and games between mother and daughter tended to minimize safe channels for the expression of aggression and sadism. Sublimation of unacceptable feelings and impulses was not facilitated by P's mother as a consistent, positive object of identification or as a role model. The attenuation of sadomasochism and hateful internalized self-object representations and relationships is greatly facilitated by mother-infant attunement and affectionate bonding rather than hostile bondage. On the other hand, P's mother's being predictably pleasant when P was compliant, and her father's affection, probably prevented more serious, suicidal psychopathology. Significant residues of caring, nurturing object and self-regard had been preserved.

Treatment Issues

A self-defeating, self-starved patient can elicit a sadomasochistic counter-transference. The analyst can feel "sucked-dry," depleted and vulnerable to feeling defeated. He/she can too readily join parent and physician in force-feeding the patient who unconsciously needs to slowly relinquish unconscious omnipotent control. The patient's negativism and masochism may foster negative therapeutic reactions and self-defeat through defeating the analyst. Masochistic acting-out may interrupt or destroy the treatment, for example, when a patient engages in substance abuse.

In life-threatening anorexia nervosa it may be necessary to use intravenous or intubated feeding until the patient is able to participate in both a supportive and dynamic psychotherapy. Supremely masochistic suicidal patients may not be appropriate for or amenable to clinical psychoanalysis. Psychoanalysis or intensive analytic psychotherapy for a mild form of anorexia nervosa without dangerous weight loss could be the treatment of choice. This would allow the anorexic patient to work through the many meanings and functions of masochistic self-starvation and to affect new modes of relating to others and attaining self-realization.

CASE II: PERVERSE MASOCHISM

Although this patient, R, a young adult male, shared some similar determinants with the previous case, the clinical picture and outcome differed. R's seeking of subjugation and humiliation was conscious, rather than disguised and unconscious, as in many other masochistic disorders such as the accident-prone personality or the gambler. His problem was a well-encapsulated, masochistic perversion dissociated from other personality traits. The term perversion is used descriptively here, shorn of judgmental connotation and stigma. He derived sexual pleasure from conscious masochistic fantasies of being dominated, humiliated, coerced, and cruelly controlled by an overpowering adult female "dominatrix." This "dominatrix" had awesome strength and determination, large breasts and prominent muscles. On occasion, she was endowed with a visible penis and once had the face of his mother. As often occurs, the perverse fantasy system was closely related to multiple perverse phenomena. This adult patient was also sexually aroused by the sight and smell of female leather jackets and shoes, particularly high heels. The dominatrix demanded total obedience and submission to any request however bizarre, disgusting, or demeaning. He was the fantasied slave of this alternating cruel and affectionate phallic woman. At times he fantasied that she demanded that he walk on all fours and bark like a dog, be spanked like a naughty child or supposedly "eat shit." His masturbation was irregularly accompanied by the utilization of pornography depicting such exciting and degrading scenarios. Unaware of his infantile demands, he had projected onto the mother figure the fantasy that "if you love me you would do anything for me." Narcissism was condensed in his victim position that required endless compensation, comfort, and consolation. I had the impression that in earlier childhood he would try to appease his mother, usually without great success. Their interaction did not fit the description of the "seduction of the aggressor" (Loewenstein, 1957). Sexual seduction of the aggressor might be one of many forms of masochistic appeasement and could actually serve adaptive avoidance of cruelty. In this formulation, the aggressor is seduced and swayed to not seriously attack through the seemingly masochistic offer or bribe of sex, money, etc., or by arousing the aggressor's sympathy, pity, shame, or guilt. Seduction of the aggressor is closely related to masochism as the weapon of the weak, to submission and appeasement to try to avoid greater sacrifice and torment.

In his young adult external behavior he chose to be socially and sexually involved with women whom he considered to be appropriate potential partners for marriage. He regarded his masochistic fantasies as weird, shameful and unacceptable. His masochistic fantasies were not obligatory for his sexual functioning and were never revealed to his fond sexual partner. He did not need to provoke his girlfriend, as he in childhood provoked his mother, to rage and rejection. Far from being a compliant "yes man." he was determined not to be timid or victimized. He could be a forceful adult in speech and manner without appearing insistent or overbearing. He was opposed to submissive appeasement, to any infringement of civil liberties and regarded himself as a true champion of the oppressed and abused. He was, in this respect, like some paranoid

personalities, on guard against any abuse of authority or power. Project-
ing an unconscious beating fantasy onto others is an important determinant in many cases of paranoia and irrational fears of attack or persecution (Freud, 1919). In reality, this patient's encapsulated perversion was
far more adaptive than the self-defeat of those masochistic characters
who are their own worst enemies in life. R was successful in school, in his
career and in his social relationships. Contrary to early psychoanalytic
assumptions, an encapsulated perversion, especially if largely confined
to fantasy, may be more adaptive than a masochistic character structure
or a self-punitive moral masochism (Blum, 1980, 2011).

Puzzled and fearful of his impulse to find a dominatrix with whom he
might act out his masochistic masturbation fantasy, R sought treatment
to insure that he maintain self-control and self-discipline. He wanted to
take charge, to be in command rather than obeying commandments. He
started analysis with ready agreement to the framework and recommendations to freely associate. He initially had an erection on the couch.
While concerned about the possible homosexual implications of his sexual arousal, he was unconsciously "submitting" to the analytic process. He
conformed to analytic requirements, and the analysis was initiated with a
perverse transference (Etchegoyen, 1991). The danger of his becoming a
"yes man" to interpretation, with unconscious fantasies of defeating the
analyst and himself, was interpreted. As the analysis evolved, the analyst
became the all-powerful, phallic, castrating and castrated dominatrix.
Unconsciously, the female dominatrix having a phallus was reassurance
against castration, but her threatening castration was not entirely alleviated. She threatened his masculinity and his "grown-up" sense of independence. The dominatrix was his sadistic alter-ego, his bisexual self, the
parental dyad and the parent-child dyad. He identified with both parents, both sexes, aggressor and victim, with unconscious ready reversal
of roles. Was he being victimized by his compliance in the analytic process, by the recumbent position (taking it lying down), the fee and the
acceptance of the authority of the analyst? Did he scan reality for possible
validations of his fantasies? Beneath an affable surface, he was all too
eager to engage in sadomasochistic power struggles. In the transference,
passive aggression changed to opposition, for example, to the framework
of time and money and to rejection of transference interpretation. As the
analysis deepened, he became increasingly aware of his psychological
warfare with his mother throughout his childhood and early adolescence.
Becoming dependent on the analyst, the transference dominatrix, he was
once impelled to partly, yet safely, enact his masochistic fantasy. He paid
for a pornographic telephone call to a menu of perverse preferences. He
chose "humiliation" and was then insulted and verbally told on the telephone that he would be punished for any insubordination. He was told
that he could not refuse to eat a dry piece of brown bread (symbolic

feces). He masturbated during the obscene phone call and afterwards was ashamed, humiliated, and filled with self-reproach.

A generally obedient child in latency, R felt entitled to sympathy rather than punishment. His infantile omnipotence was projected onto his phallic mother who provided a reality base for the projection. The patient's ambivalent relationship with her, as far as he could remember, was confirmed by his father and other relatives. His mother was "high strung" and tense, with a short temper. She could quickly withdraw affection, becoming emotionally unavailable. Intolerant of her son's aggression, she would "lock horns" and react with hostile aggression if thwarted, never taking "no" for an answer. R was informed that his mother had been rigid about his care and feeding, impatient with his crying; this paralleled the history of the anorexic patient previously discussed. R's mother seemed to feel that comforting her infant too readily would foster a spoiled child. Between his second to fourth years, R was an active, rambunctious, defiant child. Considered a "holy terror" his mother felt that she was his victim. Exasperated by his incitements, she would isolate him in his room. She was not physically abusive, but she was unmoved by his weeping, wailing protests. Like the prior patient, he too would cry until he fell asleep exhausted. In effect, she had demanded his unconditional surrender. When he awoke there would be no reference to the past battle; his mother would be affectionate and attentive, if still insensitive to his emotional states. They engaged in reciprocal, ambivalent approach and withdrawal. By the time R was in school mother and son had grown very close, especially as the relationship between his parents deteriorated. Their marital strife escalated and ultimately later they were divorced.

As time went on, R and his parents achieved a "modus vivendi." His mother, who had herself been traumatized during her first years of life during World War II and the Holocaust became less anxious. There was greater tranquility or at least an armistice while R was away during school hours. He identified with his father but was guilty about the parental divorce and his possession of his mother. However, his unconscious identification with his mother's aggression was a significant influence in his personality. Her slave in conscious masochistic fantasy, he could unconsciously coerce the object's enslavement. As a teenager, he could be sarcastic and insulting, with a well tempered sadism defending against his basic masochism. He could be despotic or dependent as master or slave, parent or child or bisexual dominatrix. In later adolescence he defended against dependent wishes as though he were refusing to submit to tyranny. Fantasied narcissistic power and glory compensated for pain and humiliation and were interwoven with his sadomasochism. R demonstrated derivatives of his mother's demand upon both him and his father for unconditional surrender. With friends, he sought dominance with his eyes in real and imagined battles to see who would "blink first." At times, he imagined people being in harmonious agreement with him but at other times in fractious discord like his parents. The visual aspect of his adolescent fantasy of the "dominatrix" was prominent and related to sadomasochistic childhood scenes. There was no evidence of primal-scene exposure, but sadomasochism had been pervasive in his pre-adult experience as well as in his fantasy life. In R's masochistic fantasy, he wrote the script, controlling the traumatic sadomasochistic situation and the punishment for pre-oedipal and oedipal transgression. In bondage and humiliation, he accepted punishment as the price of a disguised, protected childhood, reconciled with his mother. If seeking pain in fantasy preserved his feeling empowered, he could avoid being passively helpless in the face of real pain and punishment.

Significantly, the acute and extended traumas of his infancy and early childhood were the foundation of his later masochistic disposition (Novick and Novick, 1996). Mother and toddler had been "holy terrors" to each other, exacerbating the common clashes of the rapprochement phase of separation-individuation (Mahler, Pine, and Bergman, 1975). The masochistic tendencies continued through later developmental phases in his relationship with his parents, especially his mother. Mother surrogates, for example, grandmothers or maids, may have had their own additional, obscure influence. Was he addicted to pain, to the painful object (Valenstein, 1973), or were pain and humiliation amalgamated with narcissistic injury and trauma? Had trauma been erotized and at least partially transformed and narcotized with pleasurable sexual gratification? He may have been attempting to deny and undo psychic pain and suffering while simultaneously being a hidden hedonist trying to extract maximal pleasure from minimal pain. Had he adapted to protracted pain and misery through increasing tolerance for pain and frustration? At times, as a defiant youth, he seemed to anticipate being disciplined with an attitude of "grin and bear it." His erotization of punishment and trauma incorporated the narcissistic victory connected with the smile. Punishment then did not hurt, but was pleasant, with a smile denying and reversing humiliation. His masochistic telephone call was a convergence of seeking pleasure and mastering unpleasure. Far from his masochism being "Beyond the Pleasure Principle" (Freud, 1920), extracting pleasure and denying unpleasure were both features of his perverse fantasy. Punishment for forbidden oedipal wishes, and defense against castration threats, had been important developmental issues. The dominatrix having a penis provided reassurance against the threat of castration.

In the course of R's analysis his new fantasies were elaborated. Excited by televised lady wrestlers, he was intrigued by one wrestler holding the head of the other between her thighs in a scissors grip. The position of the head reminded him of birth, thus of his mother. In the transference the analyst was holding his head in a vise. He associated to scissors as a threat to excise his penis. "Scissors" evoked the phallic, castrating mother figure earlier described as the dominatrix. The two women wrestlers also represented himself identified with his mother's femininity, their quarrels, the tug-of-war between his parents. His negative oedipal complex was intensified by his flight in fantasy from the potentially castrating mother to the protective father with intact phallic genitalia. His shifting bisexual identity was also related to his shifting loyalty to one or the other parent and his serving as a messenger or arbitrator between his acrimonious parents. Unconsciously, he imagined that all three were caring or tried to symbolically castrate and humiliate each other.

The formulation of punishment because of oedipal guilt merging with masochism is a major theoretical reformulation of Freud's (1919) prior stress on sadomasochism as a vicissitude of the instinctual drives. This formulation includes the many variations on the theme of guilt and punishment in masochistic compromise formation. Punishment may be a sop to the conscience, a token punishment for achieving and enjoying orgasm. Punishment in fantasy may be temporally displaced before the oedipal transgression rather than consequent to the "crime." Acceptance of punishment beforehand may be construed as a bribe or maneuver to obtain permission, absolution or avoid greater punishment after the transgression. The balance between the guilt-ridden need for punishment and the pleasure derived from pain may vary in different cases and perhaps in different phases of life.

The quality and characteristics of the masochist's object relations is an important issue. The masochist's conscious or unconscious concern about the effect of punishment on the punitive partner must be considered. A masochistic acceptance of pain may be designed not only to arouse pity but to instill guilt in a partner via projective identification. This reversal of guilt also restores the narcissistic equilibrium of the masochist. In fantasy, the punitive partner may have been seduced into being more benign by manifest acceptance of punishment (Loewenstein, 1957). In this connection, a masochist may demonstrate a form of psychic "minimax," minimum pain for maximum gratification. This formulation is related to the acceptance of lesser punishment to escape greater punishment. Again, the over-determination of masochism encompasses varying components of punishment and narcissism as well as the affects of guilt, anxiety, humiliation, and pleasure. Unconscious guilt and the need for punishment and self-punishment may account for the close relationship of masochism to some types of depression. The fantasy of secret power in masochism is the reverse of the formulation that the masochist grants power of his life and limb to others to avoid responsibility, blame, and guilt. The unconscious power and triumph of the masochist may be disguised by manifest submission to suffering. Victory is gained through pseudo-defeat. Additionally, the masochist with a defective sense of self or an awareness of ego deficit may seek to have the dominant partner provide the needed personality functions. In more developmentally deficient or arrested personalities, masochistic pain may serve self-definition and defense against regressive loss of identity. In patients with fragile or blurred ego boundaries, masochistic surrender may represent an inviting but perilous merger. Masochistic surrender on a pre-oedipal level of development would be an impediment to separation-individuation and the consolidation of a cohesive identity. Some forms of self-cutting are simultaneously aimed at attacking the hated narcissistic object (or self-object). Insecure attachment to the primary object may be related to the "basic fault" (Balint, 1968). Pain and self-cutting may attempt to facilitate self-object differentiation as well as providing masochistic gratification and magical mastery of trauma. Suffice it to affirm that masochism may involve all levels of development and is not tied only to oedipal conflict as had been previously emphasized. Second, aggression rather than affection predominates in the more extreme forms of sadism and masochism. In parallel with the increased aggression, hatred and self-hate also dominate these extremes while love is more prominent in the mild forms of masochism and sadism. Third, extreme forms of sadomasochism are found in more highly disturbed, unstable personalities with much greater risk of serious injury to self and objects. The modulated sadomasochistic drama or game has been superceded by real, dangerous behavior.

The fantasy, and especially the reality, of being sacrificed, for example, to incest or aggressively scapegoated within the family, may be sublimated in cultural and social activities and in the guise of martyrdom. Extravagant giving and generosity may be a modified form of masochism, with repression and reversal of demands to be given to and to be over-indulged. Sublimated masochism may contribute to heroism, selflessness, and excessive humility. With sublimated aggression the sword may be beaten into the plowshare. The condensation of pain, pleasure and sexual excitement in masturbating with beating fantasies could contribute to the erotization (sexualization) of trauma. In turn, the repetition and erotization of trauma could reciprocally contribute to the mastery of pain, loss, and narcissistic injury. Pleasurable sexual stimulation may have been used to assuage pain, as likely occurred in the cited male case. Vicarious identification with the aggressor or sadist promotes the change from passive surrender to active mastery. Anna Freud (1922) in her incomplete autobiographical analysis of her own beating fantasy outlined the progressive alteration of the fantasy. Her childhood fantasy was modified in adolescence, transformed into socially acceptable stories. Masochistic pleasure gave way to pleasurable, shared social reward. These stories elicited social approval, parallel with increased self-esteem and attenuated masochism. The developmental transformation of beating fantasy has subsequently been elucidated in developmental character change.

The progressive transformation of masochistic fantasy is based on a change of aim and object, modulation of aggression, decreasing guilt and need for punishment, and the mastery of trauma. Different components of masochism may be more or less important in any individual. In addition to dynamic factors, genetic predisposition, hormonal and bodily changes, and changes in the brain as a result of trauma, illness, medication, aging, etc., may all modify masochistic fantasy and behavior. Unlike later trauma, trauma during the development of psychic structure, especially if severe and extending into subsequent phases, predisposes to severely sadomasochistic personalities. Conversely, masochists are predisposed to psychic and physical trauma through self-injury such as occurs in being accident-prone and taking perilous risks.

In contemporary psychoanalysis and neuroscience, trauma is seen as altering both the mind and brain. Trauma, inducing ego helplessness, is inevitably associated with narcissistic injury, loss of confidence and self agency. Trauma fuses narcissistic injury with increased aggression, ego regression, and developmental disturbance. The slings and arrows of later misfortune often activate earlier traumatic states with sadomasochistic accompaniment. The apparent masochistic goal of seeking pleasure in pain may be an effort to control and master trauma, intense castration and separation anxiety, and/or avoid more serious suffering and humiliation (Reik, 1941). In masochistic masturbation fantasy and enactment, revenge for, and triumph over trauma and threats from all developmental levels may be celebrated with a thrilling orgasm. No matter how injured or defeated, the orgasm proclaims the joy of survival, and intact genital function.

Castration anxiety is often prominent in male masturbation, as evident in the slang idioms of "jerk off" or "pull off." Pulling one's penis off refers to unconscious danger and in some cases to a masochistic wish. Agony may be magically converted to ecstasy. Carefully controlled regulation of pain and trauma is attempted in fantasy management of its timing, duration, and intensity. Narcissistic omnipotence is asserted in the fantasy of actively repeating trauma rather than passively enduring its recurrence. However, erotization of psychic and physical pain, trauma and traumatic anxiety are more descriptive than explanatory concepts. The psychological and possible neurobiological understanding of the erotization of trauma remains enigmatic. The fusion of sexual and aggressive drive derivatives, love and hate, as well as the fusion of pain and pleasure, may contribute to sadomasochism blended with traumatic experience. In my own clinical experience, I have considered that conditions like sexual child abuse, inevitably traumatic, or compulsive sexual activity with fantasied repetition of severe trauma, are likely determinants of the erotization of trauma. Erotized trauma is a frequent unconscious determinant of perverse masochism, but its relationship to masochistic character and to depression requires further psychoanalytic and neurobiological research.

REFERENCES

Balint, M. (1968). *The Basic Fault*. London: Tavistock.

Berliner, B. (1958). The role of object relations in moral masochism. *Psychoanalytic Quarterly* 27: 38–56.

Blos, P. (1991). Sadomasochism and the defense against recall of painful affect. *Journal of the American Psychoanalytic Association* 39: 417–30.

Blum, H. (1980). Paranoia and beating fantasy. *Journal of the American Psychoanalytic Association* 28: 331–62.

——— (1991). Sadomasochism in the psychoanalytic process; within and beyond the pleasure principle. *Journal of the American Psychoanalytic Association* 39: 431–50.

——— (2011). Masochism: Passionate pain and erotized triumph. *The Psychoanalytic Review* 98: 155–69.

Brenner, C. (1959). The masochistic character: Genesis and treatment. *Journal of the American Psychoanalytic Association* 7: 19–226.

Brody, S. (2001). *The Development of Anorexia: The Hunger Artists*. New York: International Universities press.

Cooper, A. (1988). The narcissistic-masochistic character. In *Masochism: Current Psychoanalytic Perspectives*, eds. R. A. Glick and D. I. Meyers. Hillsdale, NJ: Analytic Press, 117–38.

Etchegoyen, H. (1991). *The Fundamentals of Psychoanalytic Technique*. New York and London: Karnac Books.

Freud, A. (1922). Beating fantasies and daydreams. In *The Writings of Anna Freud, Vol. 1*. New York: International Universities Press, 137–57.

Freud, S. (1919). A child is being beaten. *Standard Edition* 17: 175–204.

——— (1920). Beyond the pleasure principle. *Standard Edition* 18: 3–64.

——— (1924). The economic problem of masochism. *Standard Edition* 19: 157–70.

Glenn, J. (1984). Psychic trauma and masochism. *Journal of the American Psychoanalytic Association* 32: 357–80.

Kucich, J. (2006). *Imperial Masochism*. Princeton, NJ: Princeton University Press.

Loewenstein R. (1957). A contribution to the psychoanalytic theory of masochism. *Journal of the American Psychoanalytic Association* 5: 197–234.

Mahler, M., Pine, F., and Bergman, A. (1975). *The Psychological Birth of the Human Infant*. New York: Basic Books.

Maleson, F. (1984). The multiple meanings of masochism in psychoanalytic discourse. *Journal of the American Psychoanalytic Association* 32: 325–56.

Novick, J., and Novick, K. (1996). *Fearful Symmetry: The Development and Treatment of Sadomasochism*. Northvale, NJ: Jason Aronson.

Parens, H. (1979). *The Development of Aggression in Early Childhood*. New York: Jason Aronson.

Reik, T. (1941). *Masochism in Modern Man*. New York: Grove Press.

Ross, J. M. (1997). *The Sadomasochism of Everyday Life*. New York: Simon & Schuster.

Valenstein, A. (1973). On attachment to painful feelings and the negative therapeutic reaction. *Psychoanalytic Study of the Child* 28: 365–92.

Winnicott, D. (1965). *The Maturational Processes and the Facilitating Environment*. New York: International Universities Press.

Zerbe, K. J. (1993). *The Body Betrayed: Women, Eating Disorders, and Treatment*. New York: American Psychiatric Press.

TEN

Failure to Thrive: Shame, Inhibition, and Masochistic Submission in Women[1]

Dianne Elise, PhD

Can you imagine how . . . it would be for our culture if women re-claimed desire?

—Shabana Azmi

Woman—does she want? If she does not, why not? If she does, what is it she wants? This question, "What does a woman want?"—possibly the central and most perplexing in the history of psychoanalysis—was almost a lament by Freud (1925), who left this quandary to female colleagues and future generations of theorists. The persistence of this question illustrates that something renders female desire opaque, both with regard to its existence and its object. Why is it not clear what women want? Some element of mystery seems to prevail; women's desire is veiled, has a hidden, shrouded quality.

The question of women's desire has generated ongoing discussion including a most cogent analysis by Benjamin (1988) that women want to want, to have a sense of agency and desire—sexual subjectivity. Dimen (1991) writes that desire is "dualistically organized, such that desire is gender syntonic for men, dystonic for women. . . . [W]omen are represented to be without desire" (p. 343)—to be the "targets" of male desire. Thus, male desire is presumed to have a clarity that stands in contrast to the seeming opacity and ambiguity of female desire. But women must have some central motive to be complicit and compliant in the myth that women lack desire (Riviere, 1929; Torok, 1970; Irigaray, 1990). What is it internally that motivates women to eclipse themselves, to accept the "si-lencing of the female first person sexual voice?" (Wolf, 1997, p. xxii).

I have proposed that the marker "absent" regarding female desire may reflect a particularly female form of defense. Whereas males may defensively *inflate*, females may *deflate*, their representation of self and desire (Elise, 2000a, 2000b). A deflated sense of subjectivity can lead to a propensity for masochistic submission. To acknowledge and actively pursue one's desire is the inverse of masochistic submission, where one subjugates one's will, one's desire, to that of the other (see Benjamin 1988). I will approach masochistic submission in women—a "failure to thrive"[2] —from the perspective of undermined female desire.

Inhibitions to female desire and an undermined sense of agency have been conceptualized within separation-individuation theory as a lack of individuation within the mother-daughter relationship. Merger has been the major lens through which to view lack of autonomy and agency in sexuality, aggression, competition, achievement, power and authority— all aspects of desire subsumed in the wish to secure relational bonds (Benjamin, 1988; Elise, 1991; Holtzman and Kulish, 2000, 2003). Clearly, multiple preoedipal determinants influence the unfolding of masochistic dynamics. My emphasis here, however, will be to highlight certain oedi-pal factors that may also play a role.

In order to delineate one particular aspect of the underlying founda-tion for masochistic submission, I want to investigate specific influences on female development at the juncture of the Oedipus complex. Through prior inquiry into the fate of the girl's oedipal wishes for her mother, I have elaborated the potential impact of an "erotic failure" that is unique to the girl (Elise, 1998a, 1998b, 2000a, 2000b, 2002, 2007, 2008). The path to heterosexual object choice determines that the girl's first erotic object choice—her mother—will not result in a "successful" oedipal pairing. I view compromised confidence regarding obtaining and keeping one's sexual love object as the heritage of what has been classically referred to as the negative oedipal complex. One result can be masochistic submis-sion—a symptomatic expression of an insecure oedipal attachment, as well as a fear of loss of love that many theorists throughout the history of the analytic literature have noted as a stronger anxiety in girls (though mainly understanding this fear in preoedipal terms). I want to directly link masochistic submission in females, as the expression of a felt need to secure relational bonds (see also Berliner, 1958), to elements of the girl's oedipal experience that I believe may heighten insecurity regarding the capacity to obtain and retain one's erotic object.

As we know, the wish to romantically win over one or both of the parents regularly meets with profound disappointment: "carried out with tragic seriousness, [it] fails shamefully . . . a permanent injury to self-regard in the form of a narcissistic scar" (Freud, 1920, pp. 20–21). It is my view that the impact of oedipal defeat, while leading to a sense of shame and inadequacy for both sexes, may result in a very different outcome for girls than for boys. It is this thesis that I will use to examine the pervasiveness of inhibition in female personality that I believe can center in sexuality and then extend to many other areas of failure to actualize desire. I hope to contribute to contemporary thinking on masochism in female psychology by elaborating the experience of oedipally based shame and by articulating what I propose as one of the many reasons that shame comes to be associated with sexuality, and especially so in females.

In order to account for inhibitions in female personality that promote dynamics of masochistic submission, I will unfold a brief developmental narrative that centers on a bodily focused narcissistic injury and sense of shame in response to unrequited erotic longings. Masochistic submission is seen from the perspective of gender-based shame that predisposes (too often) to lack of self-assertion, sexually and more generally. I will be focusing on the manner in which shame *as a female* leads to women becoming not only invested in, but often wedded to, self-destruction rather than "self-construction." Two clinical vignettes will be used to illustrate female inhibitions in agentic expression of self in sexuality, in love relationships and in professional aspirations as understood within the framework presented.

THEORETICAL FRAMEWORK

Kulish and Holtzman (1998) note the emphasis in the literature linking girls' conflicted preoedipal relationships with the mother "to later difficulties in owning and enjoying their sexuality . . . agency over sexual pleasure [is] a capacity often conflicted for many women" (p. 66). Along with other authors, Kulish and Holtzman also stress the "importance of the girl's tie to the mother in the shape, progression into or resolution of the girl's Oedipus situation" (p. 68). Rather than a struggle for power and authority seen in males, in the contrasting female oedipal story, "the maintenance of intimate relationships takes centre stage" (p. 69). In order to preserve closeness with the mother, females can defensively abdicate ownership of sexual desires, and "aggression is in the shadows" (p. 69).

It is evident that having to separate from *and compete with* the primary object is highly threatening and contributes to fear of object loss in girls. This fear of losing the (m)other fosters a prioritizing of connection to the object over responsibility to oneself for one's own impulses and wishes; such responsibility to, and for, oneself is disavowed. These female dynamics regarding separation from the object originate preoedipally and then infuse both "negative" and "positive" oedipal configurations.

Linking these two phases, Loewald (1978) underscored that: "oedipal attachments, struggles, and conflicts must be also understood as new versions of the basic union-individuation dilemma" (p. 775). Already seen earlier in the phase of separation-individuation, now oedipally an "active urge for emancipation comes to the fore" (p. 757). The mastering of the Oedipus Complex, that will take place over a lifetime, requires a wresting of authority from the parents: "By evolving our own autonomy . . . we are usurping their power, their competence, their responsibility" (p. 758). Such mastery requires a self-confidence that can only flourish when there is confidence in the relational bond.

Loewald (1978) placed strong emphasis on the need for "self-responsibility," for agentic action and autonomy rather than masochistic punishment: "Becoming independent, taking responsibility for the conduct of his own life" (p. 756) entails "appropriating parental authority" and "owning up to one's needs and impulses as one's own" (p. 761). Loewald articulated:

> [T]o develop a sense of self-identity, means to experience ourselves as agents . . . When I speak of appropriating our desires and impulses — which of course are active forces in themselves . . . I mean allowing, granting them actively that existence . . . being responsive to their urgings, acknowledging that they are ours [rather than] self-destruction . . . self-inflicted or "arranged" punishment [that] is one form of corruption. (p. 761)

In a paragraph on dynamics of submission in relation to the father in *male* development, (including identification with "mother's passive-receptive attitude toward father" (p. 760),[3] Loewald, echoing Freud, went on to remark: "If we add to this the less-well-explored intricacies of the feminine oedipal conflict, the complexities of the Oedipus complex tend to become overwhelming" (p. 760). However, Kulish and Holtzman (1998), undeterred in tracing the intricate tapestry of female development, identify that: "what is unique to the feminine positive oedipal organization derives from the fact that rivalry occurs with the same-sexed parent, the mother, who is generally the primary caretaker" (p. 68). Unique facets of female oedipal life, though complicated, can be delineated.

Pursuing this exploration, I want to lift out and disentangle the thread, not of oedipal *competition* with the mother, but of oedipal *desire for* the mother in the context of the challenging change of *erotic* object expected in the heterosexual oedipal trajectory that a girl typically traverses. The complexity of giving up her first erotic object choice is, like rivalry with the primary caretaker, unique to the girl's positive oedipal configuration. There is no parallel in boys' heterosexual development. Viewing masochistic submission in females from the vantage point of these specific "complexities" of the *feminine* oedipal conflict allows for a conceptualization of why "the assumption of responsibility for one's own life" (Loewald, 1978, p. 757) may be particularly challenging for women.

We can develop further an appreciation for why many women fail to thrive to the full extent of which they are capable.

A Gendered Fork in the Developmental Road

One sees that there is a profound difference for the two genders in the oedipal period itself. The boy gets to keep his original object—the mother—in the sense that it is at least someone of his sex that his mother wants. The boy is defeated due to his generation, not his gender. That the mother is primary caretaker (Chodorow, 1978) in preoedipal life leads to the likelihood that she will be the first oedipal object—focus of erotic desire—for *both* sexes (Freud 1931). The girl's initial confrontation with oedipal defeat is also in relation to the mother where she learns a very different lesson than does the boy: her mother does not desire someone of her sex—a gender defeat (Elise, 2000a, 2000b). She turns to the father where she then experiences the generational defeat commonly associated with the oedipal crisis (Elise, 1998b).

It is this double oedipal loss for the girl that I believe is especially significant in understanding a propensity for masochistic dynamics.[4] An experience of oedipal defeat in relation to both mother and father may leave a female with sense of inadequacy and shame that may be internalized and accepted as her identity. This outcome would contrast with a masculine phallic-omnipotent trajectory. The demise of healthy narcissism in females can underlie various expressions of pervasive inhibition and failure to actualize desire that may predispose toward masochistic submission. I suggest that girls may inhibit not only sexuality and aggression, but themselves more generally, due to a representation of self as "not having what it takes" genitally, and then psychically, to get and keep her desired love object.

Freud was clear that the first thing a girl wants is her mother. That desire is most often denied in the oedipal trajectory (Rubin, 1975; Laufer, 1986; Butler, 1990, 1995; de Lauretis, 1994; Lax, 1994, 1997). However, unlike the boy's situation, where oedipal desire for the mother is acknowledged and then forbidden, a girl's erotic desire for her mother is typically erased, negated, considered to be nonexistent (Kernberg, 1991). That a girl wants her mother is generally not seen or registered by the mother (or by anyone else). From the beginning, a girl's original experience of desire is less likely to be recognized. What she wants, and even *that* she wants, may be rendered invisible by heterosexual family structure.

Benjamin (1988) writes of the importance of mutual recognition and of the need to see the mother as a sexual subject. Both are essential to a girl's sexuality and more general expression of agentic desire. But *can the mother see the daughter* as a sexual subject? Can mother-daughter homoerotic desire be experienced and validated by the mother? The heterosexual gaze sees the boy's desire for the mother and eventually the girl's desire for the father but is typically blind to the girl's directing of these impulses and wishes toward the mother (Zak de Goldstein, 1984; Butler, 1990, 1995; Kernberg, 1991; O'Connor and Ryan, 1993; de Lauretis, 1994; Dio Bleichmar, 1995; Burch, 1997). Often, a mother has not only in concrete reality chosen a male partner, but also has internalized an assumption regarding "innate" heterosexuality and presumes erotic desire to be "naturally" a non-issue with a daughter.[5] Many analysts have shared this assumption that heterosexuality is an innate preference,[6] and thus they also assume that a girl suffers no loss in regard to her mother on an erotic level.

A girl may experience a serious defeat in her first, most intense love affair and may register this defeat as her inadequacy on a bodily level. She may come to feel that her sexed body itself is inferior (Barnett, 1966). This sense of inferiority can suffuse the entire self-representation. The oedipal loss of the father may deepen this sense of failure. Freud (1931) noted that with the girl's turn to the father and circuitous winding into femininity she relinquishes (not without a struggle) her sexuality, her desire, her activity, and her mother as love object. She stops masturbating, Freud thought. Her sexuality is permanently injured (see also Lampl-de Groot 1927). This *developmental outcome* was misconstrued in early analytic thinking to conclude that the female is "naturally" given to masochism (Deutsch, 1930; Bonaparte, 1952) and to a sense of genital inferiority as *inherent* attributes.

Freud (1931), however, noticed that something comes to a halt in female sexuality that previously was in motion: "there is to be observed a marked lowering of the active sexual impulses. . . . [T]hey have proved totally unrealizable and are therefore abandoned" (p. 239). This halt is coexistent with the turn from mother to father as primary, sexual love object, and Freud noted that this shift is unlikely to occur completely or without conflict;[7] the oedipal relation to the father inherits qualities of the original relationship with the mother. Women are often looking to re-find their mothers in their husbands: "Her relation to her mother was the original one, and her attachment to her father was built up on it, and now, in marriage, the original relationship emerges from repression. For the main content of her development to womanhood lay in the carrying over of her affective object attachments from her mother to her father" (p. 231).

Heterosexual gender role complementarity is established within the "positive" oedipal phase (Benjamin, 1988, 1995). Typically, within patriarchal family structure, when a father is present for this oedipal romance with his daughter, he is in the position of dominance (Benjamin, 1988; Butler, 1990; Elise, 1998b)—representing agency and activity. A girl's sexuality and sense of self may form as a submission to his desire. Male dominance shapes her sex into that of a passive recipient. A girl "takes refuge" (Freud, 1931) in being the passive object of the father's desire. This may be where a certain sexual "diffusivity," (see Elise, 1998b, 2000a), more general passivity, and potential for masochistic submission take root. A girl may come to feel that her body, her self and her desire are inferior to that of everyone else (Barnett, 1966). A generalized sense of impotence can ensue.

Herein lies one potential reason for females not to want: active desire might painfully revive the earliest experience of wanting and not getting the mother—never getting the mother—and of having the wrong body/ genital. If a more active wanting were to be revived, females might be in touch with wanting specific experiences first known with the mother and could experience painful disappointment and frustration in relationship to men (Dinnerstein, 1976; Chodorow, 1978; Rubin, 1983; Halberstadt-Freud, 1998). A desire to re-experience the early sensual atmosphere with the mother could appear doomed in the wished-for relationship with a man, as doomed as it generally was to retain that desire with the mother. Much is ill-fated in female sexual development: when one considers that a girl may come to experience both her body and her object choice as wrong, the impact may be significant.

Males, though, are certainly not immune from oedipal defeat and a sense of shame regarding impotent desire. A boy, however, will most typically attempt to become "big" like Dad and to make mother "small"—to triumph over her. This strategy is not a return to healthy narcissism, but a dependence on *over-inflation* of both one's genital and one's sense of self. As a corollary, mother and her female genital must be devalued. This devaluation of the female can set the stage for a masochistic-narcissistic relational pairing seen in some heterosexual couples.

While males may resort to manic inflation of their genital representation and expression of desire in hopes of immunity from an experience of castration, females—unconsciously motivated and with much support for this maneuver from the culture—may depressively and masochistically embrace the deflation of their genitals and desire (Elise, 2000a, 2000b, 2008). This feminine form of defense against being castrated (understood as in Jones's (1927) meaning of aphanisis—rendered impotent) is *parallel to, but opposite in form* from a masculine strategy of phallic omnipotence. Rather than self-promotion and aggrandizement, this feminine defensive strategy is self-defeating and belittling: masochistic. Such "protection" is based on inhibition (rather than masculine exhibition), and rests on the idea that if you *don't* "use it," (or don't [seem to] have it), you won't "lose it." A belief takes hold that it would be more shameful to try and to fail than to not try at all, and that desires are best kept as unfulfilled fantasies. Problematically for women, defensive deflation undermines one's agency, whereas inflation as a defense in activity, even if overblown, directs one out agentically into the world.

Shame as the Underside of Masochism [8]

I now want to attend more directly to the role of oedipally-derived shame as a potential determinant of masochistic submission. Freud (1933) thought of shame as a "female characteristic par excellence" (p. 132) in reaction to "genital deficiency." While I believe that males are no less vulnerable to shame at the oedipal level or to a sense of genital deficiency (Elise, 2007), the potential for feminine masochism in females is high. I am focusing specifically on the relationship of shame to libidinal drives, unrequited love, and the fate of healthy narcissism in the oedipal romance. This aspect of shame can be quite intense and may lead to long-lasting effects, particularly regarding sexuality, that are then often generalized to the entire self in gender-specific ways.

Shame—a feeling of inferiority, inadequacy, incompetence, helplessness; a sense of self as defective, flawed, leading to a pervasive sense of failure, unworthiness and to an experience of being scorned, unloved and forsaken. These are descriptions we find in psychoanalysis for what is viewed as a searing affective experience. Shame leads to a wish to hide, to keep the flawed sense of self secret and to avoid any interpersonal context that might reveal one's inadequacy and lead to further rejection (Morrison, 1989; Lansky, 2005).

Shame is a two-person experience; one is shamed in the eyes of another, even if that person is no longer literally present. At the oedipal level, shame represents the relationship of the self to another in unrequited love, an experience of lost erotic attachment to a highly cathected object. Consider the following definition by Morrison (1989): "Shame is a reflection of feelings of the whole self in failure, as *inferior in competition or in comparison* with others, as inadequate and defective" (p. 12, italics added). The experience that one has failed to capture and keep the attention, admiration, and desire of one's "significant other"—the idealized oedipal parent—leads to a belief that one's libidinal longings are unacceptable and can result in undermined or even shattered self-esteem.

Morrison (1989), following Chasseguet-Smirgel (1985), links shame with the inability to live up to the ego ideal, one's narcissism and grandiosity sinking to a sense of worthlessness and dejection and to a wish to conceal an unacceptable self. This experience of failure in relation to the ego ideal is, I believe, regularly and normatively triggered by the oedipal object(s) being unattainable, understood by the child as a failure due to defect in the self—being small, inadequate—literally "falling short."

The would-be oedipal contender is "pumped up and ready to go," only to find little or no reciprocal, affirming response to these desires. Both sexes are forced to contend with a big/little polarity that now has sharp consequences regarding one's sexual body and romantic aspirations. The oedipal child is left to deflate; there is nowhere to go but down. Children feel shamed, and often are shamed, for "thinking big" romantically and erotically and then being exposed inevitably as little—not a contender.[9]

Schalin (1989) detailed the positive versus defensive nature of phallic narcissism in both sexes. Healthy exhibitionistic expression of phallic intention takes the form of wanting to make a positive impression upon another person. There is an advantage to making explicit the tumescence of genital and mind—the exhibitionistic glee—that is conveyed in phallic narcissism. As Freud believed girls could be phallic, I think he was identifying a quality of sexual self-experience that is essential in understanding the contrasting experience: how shame comes to be so attached to sex (and that Freud did connect to girls' sense of genital inadequacy and departure from sexuality). A concept of healthy inflation needs to be accessible in order to appreciate a problematic sense of deflation. Then we can more fully account for the wide extent of narcissistic injury that shows up regarding the sexual body and then sex, itself. I am not sure that psychoanalysis has ever adequately theorized healthy genital exhibitionism for girls.

Bernstein (1990) argued that: "the girl's body, her experiences with it and conflicts about it are as central to her development as the boy's body is to his"" (p. 152). I have proposed (Elise, 1997) that we use the phrase "primary sense of femaleness" in order to highlight early bodily awareness—a bodily sense of self that corresponds to the sexed body one inhabits as a female (see also Kulish, 2000). For boys, genital feeling is sensed as emanating out from the body, the most intense pleasure a few inches out from the torso. In holding the penis, they feel its extension outward, somewhat separable from the rest of the body. Girls locate both a feeling and an organ that is flush with, and infusing, the torso and that seems to have some inner potential (Mayer, 1985; Tyson, 1994). Both sexes begin life with an inherent sense of genital sufficiency.

Sensate experience of one's genital structure has the capacity to lend shape to one's ego—to make particularly salient certain configurations as a sort of internal mapping of the body, the self, and the world. It is obvious that the sexism of the culture has privileged phallic intention—linearity, following the straight and narrow, expansion into the world and penetration of outer space. Women have often been viewed as wandering around in circles, not having a straightforward view of situations, and of getting nowhere fast. This devaluation of women is internalized by women, extending into masochistic trends in relating as a gendered dynamic that, while not limited to women, is prominent in female psychology.

As I have emphasized, for both sexes shame attached to oedipal defeat is almost unavoidable developmentally. The infantile nature of oedipal sexuality lends itself to an experience of shame as a frequent element of the human sexual condition and gives rise to a wish to hide from exposure. The gaze of the other and the visual image of the self become highly charged territory abounding with anxieties about how one is viewed, both concretely and symbolically. For each sex, oedipal defeat means that the gendered ego ideal is not realized, but how the two sexes typically contend with such shame tends generally to follow very different trajectories.

Women, as a sex, often tend to be more on sexual display. Looking and being looked at also tend to break down into gendered divisions along the lines of an active subject and a passive object (see Dio Bleichmar, 1995). Women as the objects of male sexual gazing are often passively, anxiously, even masochistically on exhibit rather than more actively and confidently exhibitionistic. As sexual anxieties and insecurities tend to become gender specific in their shaping, so too, do defenses: men more likely turn passive into active, while too often women seem to sink into an acceptance of shame, a need to hide and/or masochistic submission. A feminine devaluation of self combines with a heightened fear of, and anxious focus on, object loss, here understood as loss of the object's desire.

CLINICAL ILLUSTRATIONS

In the Gaze of the (M)Other

I will now offer case material from an analysis of a female patient that illustrates a pronounced, though not rare, sense of shame regarding sex, an image of herself as inadequately small, and an inhibition, repudiation, even repulsion toward active female desire. These dynamics are not overtly masochistic in the more pathological sense but reflect a fairly common feminine diminishment of self that expresses submission to a relinquishment of pleasure in favor of maintaining an object relationship. Of course, these dynamics are complexly determined, but I am highlighting the potential influence, tucked away in an erotic relationship to a man, of the oedipally desired maternal object.

Consider the following session with Sara who, after a few years in analysis, arrives uncharacteristically late:

P: I'm late today because I want to bring up a new topic. Well, I want to talk about it, but, then again, I don't. It's about sex.

When I ask her what had made it difficult to bring sex up earlier in our work, she at first denies the subject's importance to her. But then she acknowledges how she has avoided — even hidden — her concerns by occasional and seemingly comfortable references to sex designed to put me "off the track." She then confesses a preference for masturbation over sex with her husband.

P: I feel a freedom masturbating; it's all mine; I can fantasize whatever I want with no concern about someone else. By myself, no one can see me. I fantasize about myself when I was younger and more attractive. Orgasm is so reliable in masturbating, but with my husband it's not.

It feels like sex is for him, and masturbation is for me. I have to talk myself into sex with him. When it's just me, I feel that urge and just go for it.

Noting that she had avoided any specifics about her body, I inquire. Sara painfully catalogues bodily "defects."

P: I wouldn't do cosmetic surgery, but there isn't a week that goes by that I don't think, fix these (she gestures to her eyelids), lift these (breasts), erase these stretch marks (belly). . . . In my fantasies, my body looks great. I've spent a lot of time feeling I'm supposed to *love* sex, be super sexy in bed, be a fabulous experience for the guy. But it doesn't lead to orgasm for me; I'm always so focused on what I can do for him, being sexually superlative; it's all an act."

I respond:

A: All this effort to be pleasing interferes with focusing on your own pleasure.

She agrees. Although men seemed very pleased with Sara as a sex partner, her sexy self is a persona, one that gives her narcissistic gratification but not much bodily pleasure. The need for self-esteem and securing the relationship trumps sexual gratification—a trade too frequently made by women.

Sara conveys to me that her focus on the man's pleasure includes her preoccupation with *his* pleasure at her having a perfect, young body. In masturbatory fantasies, she can arrange this scenario with elements involving sexy lingerie and orchestrated sexual positions. In actual sex, her husband does not necessarily arrange the scene to create the sexy visual of her body, so she experiences sex as the context in which her flaws are exposed, and she wants to avoid this shame. In our exchanges, the symbolic exposure to me of her flawed body/self furthers, in the transference, Sara's sense of shame, deficiency, and inadequacy. Just how long she had delayed discussion of this topic, when it was regularly on her mind, is significant regarding the vulnerability to a sense of sexual shame even in relation to another woman. Note that sex as a topic had not been markedly absent in a way that would typically alert an analyst. Periodic mention, references to sex and description of some dissatisfaction with marital sex life had obscured the fact that the real issues had "slipped under the radar."

After our initial foray into this shame-infused realm, a massive avoidance set in that was difficult to alleviate, and that proved to be, session after session, a rather impenetrable obstacle to attempts on my part to link back to what had been revealed. Sara recounted a trip to the zoo as a girl:

P: Two animals mated, the male mounted, the female seemed stuck there, trapped, looking both degraded and bored.

In addition to being a rather grim, masochistic image of female sexuality, this association seemed to depict her feeling in the transference.

As I continued to identify how the experience of shame led to a feeling that avoidance was the best option, she did eventually reopen the topic:

P: My friend Kim is overweight and rather pear-shaped; she looks way better with her clothes on, but she seems to feel fine about herself.

A: How do you understand that—her not being critical of her imperfect body?

P: I guess she doesn't have the same standards I do for myself.

A: Why do you think you have them?

P: That's the six-million-dollar question, isn't it?" (pause).

A: Something leads to a sense of your being under the shadow of this impossible standard. And you are not actually in your body or experiencing the immediacy of a sexual encounter. You are outside, observing, listing flaws and judging yourself as inadequate, not worth much, not worthy of pleasure, submitting for the sake of the man's pleasure. Flaws are a cause for rejection. Fear of rejection leads to a vulnerable, anxious focus on flaws and a need to hide them."

P: I can't imagine someone not being critical of my bodily flaws; if they look and see imperfections, it's ugly, not sexy . . . (long pause). With one man I did have great sex; I felt totally free. And accepted.

A: What do you think made the difference?

P: I sensed how much he cared for me. During sex he looked straight into my eyes with an intense feeling of connection.

A: That close eye contact reassured you he wasn't standing back scanning you for flaws—evaluating, assessing, judging, criticizing.

P: It's not that the men I've been with have actually done that; no one has that I can think of . . . (extended pause) well, my mother . . . [Sara gives numerous examples from girlhood of adoring her mother, yet feeling physically scrutinized by her in a way that made her feel "small."] I felt . . . well, not quite right, dismissed somehow. And then in my later puberty development, I really *was* small—the little skinny one, with two bumps on my chest, knock-kneed; I didn't think I was ever gonna be a woman. Other girls were voluptuous, wearing grown up women's shoes. I was wearing kiddy shoes; my feet were so small. It was really a challenge to find sophisticated clothing and shoes because back then kids stuff was really kids stuff. My mother seemed sympathetic, but she couldn't really relate; she was so beautiful and full-figured. Some guys thought I was "cute," but cute seemed little, diminished, not sexy. When I did see guys looking at my body, I guess I thought I had finally filled out and wasn't the scrawny little kid anymore.

A: Something in the way you registered your own body seemed to block the knowledge that you'd filled out until the gaze of others really communicated this new sense of yourself to you.

There was no mention of Sara's father in this material (though it can be assumed that the paternal oedipal relation was influenced by, and influenced, the maternal oedipal experience). Sara seemed preoccupied with a sense of gendered inadequacy in relation to her mother but not in the standard formulation of oedipal competition for the father. Instead, Sara's desire to show up—"fill out"—in *the gaze of her mother* seemed central.

Eventually, Sara revealed fantasies of being seduced, overpowered, wishing not to be responsible for her own sexuality. I ask her what it means to be responsible.

P: When I think about women being turned on—I can hardly say the word "horny"—I'm repelled. When Kim says she got "wet," it makes me cringe. Any bodily evidence of being turned on, "wanting it" is repulsive. Men can take off sexually on their own. You could be "dead" underneath them and they can carry on, come, and feel just fine about themselves. But as a woman, no matter how jazzed you are, if you get all carried away, well, the man can "drop out" and you just can't keep on going without him/his excitement. You're left high and . . . well, I was gonna say, high and dry, but actually it's worse—

you're left high and wet! They should change that saying. Something about being the only one feeling horny seems shameful, degraded, for a woman, like you're ridiculous to be all "hot and bothered"—now there's a saying we can keep! A woman alone in lust is a subject of ridicule, humiliated; a man, a proud phallic animal looking for a conquest.

(End of session.)

Due to a sense of shame, Sara inhibits her own desire and "submits" to a sexual relationship with her husband that is not sadomasochistic in the usual sense but that does involve psychic masochism in the giving up on the pursuit of direct sexual pleasure for herself. The relinquishment of pleasure (sexual fulfillment) in exactly the place one expects to find it can be quite psychically painful, even if in a dull, deadening manner.

Kulish and Holtzman (1998) speak of women's "greater inhibition in the ability to take responsibility for their sexuality" (p. 66); they explicate through the Persephone myth a tendency in women to view sexuality as something forced upon them and from which it is difficult to escape. To take responsibility sexually means being willing to validate one's own pursuit of pleasure rather than having the sole aim of pleasing the other. The prospect of not pleasing a man gets right to the heart of a fear of object loss with explicit links to oedipal defeat that, as I have indicated, is likely a redoubled experience for girls. Paraphrasing Freud (1893) regarding normative unhappiness, we might think of the common masochism of everyday life that often goes "under the radar" in women's sexual relationships. Women can foreclose their potential to be potent sexually, and as a person.

Anxiety associated with "sticking out" may especially pertain to women's, not solely to men's, wish for (genital) potency. Concern about failing to engage, or out-stripping, the male libido, can wither female libido. Yet, oedipally, it is *female* libido—the mother's—that the girl likely fails to engage. Rather than being embedded in a reciprocal, erotic, oedipal relation with her mother, a girl is too often left alone without a partner. What may be "cut off" for the girl, in encountering the reality of unrequited oedipal desires, is her self-esteem regarding her genitals as well as her sense of (sexual) potency and prowess. How clinicians hold these ideas in mind, especially in considering an oedipally derived, gendered sense of shame as a substrate of masochistic submission, makes a significant difference in how one hears and works with analytic material.

The Trophy Husband

With the next patient I will present, masochistic submission is more evident throughout the entirety of the couple's dynamics. Yet once again, shame, a devalued sense of self and fear of object loss lead to inhibition and submission rather than agentic assertion and self-responsibility. A sense of oedipal failure is reiterated in the marriage and proves difficult to work through. Again, erotic defeat in relation to the maternal object can be seen to subtly infuse the heterosexual relationship.

Kate has seen her husband as superior to her in almost every way, admiring him and feeling deficient herself. In reality, her husband is exceedingly narcissistic and much less mature than Kate. The idealization that had her thinking of him as a "good catch" has been slowly giving way in the analysis, and Kate is starting to question the basis for her feelings of intimidation:

P: I realize how really scared I am to assert what I want in my marriage and professionally as well. I see that I believe I can't get the kind of mature relationship that I want because I'm not that mature myself.

She speaks of her emotional reactivity and volatility.

A: What is it that compels your emotional reactivity?

P: A lack of ground under me: when I'm able to move from a more mature place in myself, it comes from a sense of having a ground under me.

Kate gives some examples of maturity in her parenting:

P: I see that I have maturity *there* that I don't usually recognize in myself more generally.

A: Through misrecognition, or even an erasure, of your strengths, you're not making full use of your maturity.

P: Yes . . . now I'm pulled back into my childhood: I was much younger than my sisters, but I felt from an early age that I was *more* mature—"older."

We discuss how Kate needed to disavow her maturity, especially as her parents seemed quite immature themselves; she jettisoned her mature aspects in order to bolster her objects so that she could have a sense of relating to "strong" people. This masochistic submission— *being "less than" in order to be with*—has left her feeling that she has nothing to offer to someone she would actually think of as a healthy match.

P: I feel like a nobody—just floating around in the universe.

I ask how as a child Kate held her sense of being more mature than her family members *and* like a nobody.

P: When I'd look in the mirror as a kid, I saw myself as ugly, incredibly ugly. For a long time I saw this as a fact, not just a feeling state—a fact. Everyone could see it.

A: Your ugly view of yourself matched how you felt mirrored by your parents and older sisters.

P: This all goes along with my feeling of being vulnerable: stupid, ugly and embarrassingly young—"a dirty puddle." It's not good to show vulnerability.

A: Can you say more about what it means to you to be young and vulnerable?

P: You wouldn't want to be partnered with me; it would be a total embarrassment to you if anyone knew you and I were together.

A: In what ways would I be embarrassed?

P: The fact that I was clinging onto you—the opposite of a "trophy wife"—a small ball of snot.

A: A tiny little girl wanting to be close, to be together, with her mother. This little girl who wants to "cling on" feels stupid, ugly and embarrassingly young/vulnerable, not at all desirable.

P: I'm thinking about the qualities I'd want in a partner/friend; I realize how I go after 'trophy' relationships so I'll look better; I do this with Tom (her husband). He's great and he's *with me*.

I speak to her about how her pairing up with a trophy spouse does not actually "transfer" these wished for qualities to her "ugly" self but instead further drains her agentic sense of self. Kate has sought a borrowed self-esteem by relational proximity that has actually undermined her sense of self worth:

A: In fact, the more mature qualities that you do possess are obscured from view, kept unrecognized and underdeveloped. You continue to look in the mirror and misrecognize yourself, seeing yourself as without resources of your own that you can appreciate and develop.

P: What am I afraid of? What the hell keeps me doing this? I'm not feeling self-accusatory, just feeling the impact of how persistent this all is. . . . I don't know why, but I'm thinking about a TV show about Dracula that my daughter was watching.

A: Any thoughts about that?

P: Blood suckers . . . (extended pause).

A: Vampires live off the blood of others left drained of vitality, limping along soon to be the "undead." Yet, the ingénue "victim" initially sees Dracula as powerful and erotically compelling—a trophy husband.

Kate and I both laugh.

A: But the desire to submit to, in order to unite with, his power actually drains her of any strength.

P: (after a long pause) I can keep alive—less sucked on—if I pretend I'm already dead. He will never let me go. This dynamic—toxic and sickening—is so huge inside me, it would take an exorcism or a blood transfusion. It's so deeply rooted—I see it, but I can't let go of it.

The Dracula theme is used to see the "tie" as an internal dynamic from which it is difficult to extricate herself without external help (nutrition/analysis).

A: You would have to be ready to go forward on your own strength; that's a lot to be ready for. . . . We need to stop.

P: I just had this unusual, strange thought about the session: Did I do this right?

Kate sounds doubtful.

One can see in this material the mother-daughter erotic relation reflected in an expression of erotic transference where Kate feels not just little and (sexually) inadequate but completely ugly, stupid, and repellent ("snot"). In the progression of the analysis, depleted self-esteem had become evident in the transference as Kate began to contact erotic wishes to be partnered with the analyst. The sense of shame and inadequacy showed up in relation to me as an inhibition in elaborating her libidinal longings for a maternal oedipal figure (to be close to me erotically, as well as more generally). Erotic transference wishes could be referred to but resisted deeper elaboration and were most often diluted or circumvented in being split off to objects outside the analytic dyad. As Kate once expressed: "What would be the point of going into these feelings? I'd just be stuck."

She imagined that expression of these erotic wishes would lead to a masochistic submission to her analyst that would result in a stasis (like her marriage) and deplete her, obviating analytic progress. However, as seen in this session, Kate does have the growing belief that she has maturity in certain areas, and that she might recognize and further develop her strengths in her own right rather than by relational submission to a trophy husband, attempting to borrow strength by proximity (narcissistic extension).

The image of Dracula as the ultimate trophy husband—handsome, powerful, vigorous (as he enters the scene in various films)—captures the marital dynamic Kate is embroiled in, her need to idealize interwoven with her husband's narcissistic issues. The relationship bedevils her, maintaining an addictive lure from which it is very hard to separate and individuate, as she is even further depleted of nutritious narcissistic supplies ("blood"). She sees herself as having few internal resources that would sustain her; thus, maturing and individuating from an oedipal dynamic of submission feels impossible. Just as in films, for the blood-sucked victim to free herself from Dracula always takes incredible force and the efforts of many in order to "save" the woman from erotic enthrallment.

This vampire representation of a sadomasochistic relationship, both sexually and more generally, is recognizable as a familiar feminine, romantic fantasy. The iconic Dracula tale parallels themes in the Persephone myth but with erotic enthrallment and masochistic submission highlighted. For Loewald (1978), such a "romance" would represent a failure to work through the passive-submissive attachment to the oedipal object toward a more mature, individuated object relationship.

The Dracula theme provides a metaphor for dynamics, both preoedipal and oedipal, of narcissistic supply and loss in the self vis-à-vis a hungry object; the hungry self is wedded to an object even hungrier than the self. Can masochistic submission be understood apart from wounded narcissism in self and other? If a girl is not fed enough narcissistic supplies in the mother-daughter relationship (including, and maybe even *especially*, in the early oedipal situation), then she is likely to be vulnerable to relating to a (potentially narcissistic) oedipal figure in masochistic submission. In an adult relationship where it is difficult to be clear who is feeding off of whom, a masochistic-narcissistic union—a particular form of pair-bonding—continues to deplete a healthy narcissistic investment in the development of self. Individuation is a relational threat in the masochistic-narcissistic couple.

To go in the direction of the developing self is believed to be at the cost of maintaining the tie to the narcissistic oedipal (as well as preoedipal) object (which it may well be if the real life partner can not mature as well). An object relation of masochistic submission is internalized so as to avoid the other's narcissistic injury and retaliatory rejection. One either submits or loses the connection/attachment. One loses either way, but submission keeps the object relation in place. With a partner whose fragility and potential for narcissistic injury is high, submission cannot be refused without a breach in the relational "security."

To strike out "on one's own" feels as if it means "going solo" indefinitely, which feels intolerable, especially with a weakened sense of self. This emotional situation has resonances with what a child would have to surmount in deciding it is necessary to leave home—not a choice most children could make. Instead, one most likely attempts to make do with a bad situation, continuing to subsist on relational malnutrition, getting weaker and weaker, unless "supplies" can be located from some source external to the primary bond. Yet since the nature of such a relationship ensures limited development of external supports, often both personally and professionally, extricating oneself can be very challenging.

FEMININE MASOCHISM IN FEMALES

> Freud . . . for his theory of development the important thing was to get the girl to *become feminine* and ready to receive love and babies passively from an active man. (Schafer, 1974, p. 477, italics added)

Masochism can be viewed as a disorder of desire. I have conceptualized masochistic submission as a relinquishment of one's own desire, motivated by a fear of object loss. Shame and a depleted sense of self-worth, derived from or intensified by oedipal defeat, lead to inhibiting one's own desire, trying instead to fulfill the desire of the other and typically failing to do so. Without "self-construction," self-destructive actions or inactions predominate.

I have proposed that a girl's experience that, because she is a girl, the first oedipal object—her mother—is not "accessible" now or later, may play its own specific role in generating a relational strategy of masochistic submission as a fearful "grasp" on the object. Oedipal failure for the girl qua girl in relation to the mother as first erotic object choice begins her heterosexual journey: the expected turn to the father occurs at the site of her failure to "win" her mother. In relation to first the mother, then the father, active frequently turns to passive, and "femininity" as a relational strategy sets in and takes hold. One *becomes* feminine.[10]

We have long known (Broverman et al., 1970) that the stereotypic characteristics of femininity (passive, timid, coy, pleasing, docile, submissive, dependent, etc.) align with masochism (see Elise, 1997). These gendered traits, not far removed from masochism, led Freud (1924) to identify the second of his three forms of masochism as "feminine masochism." Freud was analyzing "feminine" masochism in males, making it evident that feminine masochism is not inherently female; something has to account for its development in males *and in females*. I suggest that if fathers were to have been the primary caretakers, Freud's second formulation would have been "masculine masochism." Additionally, each of my thesis points would then apply in reverse to male development: oedipal failure with the father, as first erotic object, would lead to a boy's gendered, bodily sense of inadequacy and undermined confidence in obtaining a desired love object.

Steyn (2009) asks: "Is feminine masochism a concept worth reviving?" (p. 867) and answers in the affirmative. I concur with Steyn that this term can be usefully employed, that it signals a specific defense in flight from oedipal sexual conflicts, and that careful attention needs to be paid to the word "feminine." The intent is not to convey a basic assumption that masochism is inherent in female nature but instead to refer to a masochistic position taken up (by females or by males) that aligns with a culturally entrenched gender role internalized at a very deep level through early object relations. Feminine masochism is a maneuver enacted for purposes of defense against oedipal anxieties. The specific anxiety that I am addressing is the fear of not getting, or of losing, the object's desire.

In discussing male development, Steyn (2009) notes that a mother who discourages separation and differentiation "encourages a feminine development," (p. 871) that undermines sexual desire and assertion in the child.[11] She continues: "What Freud described in feminine masochism was the way in which a certain identificatory position was adopted to stunt development out of anxiety" (p. 872). I suggest that this conceptualization might be productively applied to a *girl's* (as well as a boy's) flight from sexual desire, individuation, and agency. Girls, too, can employ femininity in the service of defense against oedipal anxieties that include fears of narcissistic injury, impotence and rejection.

Marital Dynamics

In looking at masochistic submission in adult couples, one sees that the internal object worlds of two individuals intertwine. Sara and Kate each *interpreted* their relationship with their husband to *require* a submissive stance sexually and more generally. Most likely they each paired with a man who actively contributed to this dynamic. Female masochism easily resides with male narcissism. Even so, neither woman was able to use her considerable communication skills and relational capacities to the advantage of herself, her husband or the marital bond. Instead, both Sara and Kate continued the internalized parental object relation that led them to feel inadequate sexually, interpersonally and in aspects of life outside the marriage. In tandem with masochistic submission to a narcissistic husband, these women, like many others, have encountered significant inhibitions in their work life (see Applegarth, 1976). The inhibition of professional development then returns them to, and reinforces, a submissive stance in relation to the husband. The marriage becomes a "declaration of dependence" (Symonds, 1971).

With these and several other women patients I have treated, masochistic submission as a particular marital dynamic served to reinforce on multiple levels varying degrees of overt masochism in each of the women. Instead of thinking in terms of a sadomasochistic pairing, I am discussing what might be thought of as a maso-narcissistic union. This conceptualization allows for thinking about female masochistic submission in couples without attributing to the partners the pathological extent that the term sadism usually connotes. A "failure-to-thrive" dynamic was evident in each of these women and was a clinically useful conceptual model—organizing treatment and an interpretive approach—able to be directly communicated to patients without being taken as condemnation. To articulate, understand and work through obstacles to thriving fostered oedipal individuation in each woman and an ability to "stand on her own" *within* a healthier marital context. Helping women (and men) to extricate themselves from these restrictive dynamics that inhibit both the individual self and the health of pair-bonding, facilitates increasingly mature development.

In writing about maturing object relations, Loewald (1978) emphasized:

> In the process of becoming and being an adult, significant emotional ties with parents are severed . . . a form of taking over actively what had to be endured passively in the beginning (p. 756). What will be left if things go well is tenderness, mutual trust, and respect—the signs of equality . . . [whereas evasion] is a way of preserving libidinal-dependent ties (p. 758). In mature object relations . . . the self engages, in a return movement as it were, with objects that are differently organized . . . [leading to] novel ways of relating with objects . . . a sea-change on the plane of object love. (p. 763)

When such transformations do not occur, repetitive oedipal dynamics are reiterated, impeding the creative process needed to achieve novel resolutions.

In wanting a relationship with a man, women are pressed, not solely by a partner but more importantly, by internalized cultural expectations insinuated into marital dynamics, to shape the relationship and themselves in a particular way. Both men and women are inducted into these polarized roles of male dominance and female submission and accommodation through the internalization of early object relations (Benjamin 1988). Given these cultural and familial expectations, full recognition and expression of women's desire can threaten this highly valued love relationship for women; thus, women may backpedal on one form of desire (assertion of self) to achieve another (relational "security"), often finding themselves in a masochistic trap of growing proportions. This strategy is a manifestation of the need in men and women alike to see the male as superior. Female desire poses a threat to the power balance accepted and expected in a paternalistic culture regarding heterosexual gender roles (Chasseguet-Smirgel, 1976; Person, 1980; Benjamin, 1988; Johnson, 1988). A woman's sexuality, and more general agentic expression of self, cannot come into its own while its expression is felt to threaten the attainment of a desired love bond with a man.

CONCLUSION

I have proposed that oedipal defeat in relation to either parent can result in a narcissistic injury—a "castration"—that originates as a gendered as well as a generational experience. A sense of disappointment and deflation may ensue regarding one's sexed body and one's romantic aspirations. For females, living out a dejected, deflated stance (classically understood in a limited way as penis envy) sends them in the direction of a continued sense of shame, inhibition, and masochistic relational tendencies. In the derailment of female desires, being "small" may become a way of life.

Lerner (1976) famously pointed out that the lack of adequate information given to the girl regarding her sexual body often leads to anxiety, confusion, and shame regarding her sexuality. I hope to have conveyed that a "laying low" of female sexual agency is a microcosm of more general trends in female personality: anxiety, ambivalence, and inhibition regarding agency, aggression, competition, envy, power, achievement, and authority—basically any form of self-assertion.We know that these attributes are needed in many life pursuits—professional ambitions, creative endeavors, athletic prowess, etc. Yet, multiple determinants of a submissive stance are deeply embedded within the object relational world. Recognition of these complex developmental factors, located within the object relational matrix, that contribute to submission in females illuminates more fully how female inhibitions, though often railed against by women themselves, can become so masochistically entrenched.

NOTES

1. This chapter draws on material from two previously published papers (Elise, 2000, 2008).

2. I am borrowing the phrase used when infants do not grow in a robust manner.

3. Note that throughout the analytic literature, a *girl's* identification with a mother's passive-receptive attitude toward father is often thought to be unproblematic.

4. Of course, females (and males) vary immensely in any individual propensity for masochistic submission. Complex factors that contribute to, or help work against,

masochistic submission are multiply layered and will find unique expression in any given person.

5. Certainly, when a mother does recognize and respond in an affirming manner to her daughter's erotic energy, such support helps greatly to attenuate oedipal injury. It still would be a delicate task to deal with the blow to a daughter's narcissism, and to her desire for her mother, dealt by the mother's choice of a male partner.

6. An assumption of heterosexuality as innate neglects the centrality of psychic bisexuality in Freud's oeuvre, as well as in the unfolding psychoanalytic literature.

7. See Harris (1991) for a famous case in point.

8. I am extending the title of Morrison's (1989) classic text in suggesting that shame is the underside of masochism (as well as of narcissism).

9. When an oedipal child is "let down" gently, parental counter-balancing support to self-esteem can make a significant difference in ameliorating shame-inducing aspects of oedipal defeat. The presence or absence of such support accounts for individual variations in coming to terms with a normative developmental challenge.

10. Getting a girl to become feminine was not merely a conceptual strategy in Freud's theoretical model; Freud was describing something that he observed in female development and that has been famously depicted by De Beauvoir (1952).

11. See Torok (1970) and Elise (1991) for an analysis of this dynamic in the mother-daughter relationship.

REFERENCES

Applegarth, A. (1976). Some observations on work inhibitions in women. *Journal of the American Psychoanalytic Association* 24S: 251–68.

Barnett, M. (1966). Vaginal awareness in the infancy and childhood of girls. *Journal of the American Psychoanalytic Association* 14: 29–141.

Benjamin, J. (1988). *The Bonds of Love*. New York: Pantheon.

——— (1995). *Like Subjects, Love Objects*. New Haven, CT: Yale University Press.

Berliner, B. (1958). The role of object relations in moral masochism. *The Psychoanalytic Quarterly* 27: 38–56.

Bernstein, D. (1990). Female genital anxiety, conflicts and typical mastery modes. *International Journal of Psychoanalysis* 71: 151–65.

Bonaparte, M. (1952). Some biopsychical aspects of sado-masochism. *International Journal of Psychoanalysis* 33: 373–84.

Broverman, I. K., Broverman, D. M., Clarkman, F. E., Rosencrantz, P. S., and Vogel, S. R. (1970). Sex role stereotypes and clinical judgements of mental health. *Journal of Consulting and Clinical Psychology* 34: 1–7.

Burch, B. (1997). *Other Women: Lesbian/bisexual Experience and Psychoanalytic Views of Women*. New York: Columbia University Press.

Butler, J. (1990). *Gender Trouble: Feminism and the Subversion of Identity*. New York: Routledge.

——— (1995). Melancholy gender: Refused identification. *Psychoanalytic Dialogues* 5: 165–80.

Chasseguet-Smirgel, J. (1976). Freud and female sexuality: The consideration of some blind spots in the exploration of the "Dark Continent." *International Journal of Psychoanalysis* 57: 275–86.

——— (1985). *The Ego Ideal*. New York: Norton.

Chodorow, N. (1978). *The Reproduction of Mothering*. Berkeley: University of California Press.

De Beauvoir, S. (1952). *The Second Sex*. New York: Alfred A. Knopf, Inc.

De Lauretis, T. (1994). *The Practice of Love*. Bloomington: Indiana University Press.

Deutsch, H. (1930). The significance of masochism in the mental life of women. *International Journal of Psychoanalysis* 11: 48–60.

Dimen, M. (1991). Deconstructing difference: Gender, splitting, and transitional space. *Psychoanalytic Dialogues* 1: 335–52.

Dinnerstein, D. (1976). *The Mermaid and the Minotaur*. New York: Harper & Row.

Dio Bleichmar, E. (1995). The secret in the constitution of female sexuality: The effects of the adult's sexual look upon the subjectivity of the girl. *Journal of Clinical Psychoanalysis* 4: 331–42.

Elise, D. (1991). An analysis of gender differences in separation-individuation. *The Psychoanalytic Study of the Child* 46: 51–67.

———— (1997). Primary femininity, bisexuality and the female ego ideal: A re-examination of female developmental theory. *The Psychoanalytic Quarterly* 66: 489–517.

———— (1998a). Gender repertoire: Body, mind and bisexuality. *Psychoanalytic Dialogues* 8: 353–71.

———— (1998b). The absence of the paternal penis. *Journal of the American Psychoanalytic Association* 46: 413–42.

———— (2000a). Woman and desire: Why women may not want to want. *Studies in Gender & Sexuality* 1: 125–45.

———— (2000b). Generating gender: Response to Harris. *Studies in Gender & Sexuality* 1: 157–65.

———— (2002). Blocked creativity and inhibited erotic transference. *Studies in Gender & Sexuality* 3: 161–95.

———— (2007). The Black man and the mermaid: Desire and disruption in the analytic dyad. *Psychoanalytic Dialogues* 17: 791–809.

———— (2008). Sex and shame: The inhibition of female desires. *Journal of the American Psychoanalytic Association* 56: 73–98.

Freud, S. (1893). The psychotherapy of hysteria from studies on hysteria. *Standard Edition* 2: 253–305.

———— (1920). Beyond the pleasure principle. *Standard Edition* 18: 1–64.

———— (1924). The economic problem of masochism. *Standard Edition* 19: 157–70.

———— (1925). Some psychical consequences of the anatomical distinction between the sexes. *Standard Edition* 19: 248–58.

———— (1931). Female sexuality. *Standard Edition* 21: 221–44.

———— (1933). New introductory lectures on psychoanalysis: Femininity. *Standard Edition* 22: 112–35.

Halberstadt-Freud, H. (1998). Electra versus Oedipus: Femininity reconsidered. *International Journal of Psychoanalysis* 79: 41–56.

Harris, A. (1991). Gender as contradiction. *Psychoanalytic Dialogues* 1: 197–224.

Holtzman, D., and Kulish, N. (2000). The feminization of the female oedipal complex, Part I: A reconsideration of the significance of separation issues. *Journal of the American Psychoanalytic Association* 48: 1413–37.

———— (2003). The feminization of the female oedipal complex, Part II: Aggression reconsidered. *Journal of the American Psychoanalytic Association* 51: 1127–51.

Irigaray, L. (1990). This sex which is not one. In *Essential Papers on the Psychology of Women*, ed. C. Zanardi. New York: New York University Press.

Johnson, M. (1988). *Strong Mothers, Weak Wives*. Berkeley: University of California Press.

Jones, E. (1927). The early development of female sexuality. In *Papers on Psychoanalysis*. Boston: Beacon Press, 1961, 459–72.

Kernberg, O. (1991). Sadomasochism, sexual excitement, and perversion. *Journal of the American Psychoanalytic Association* 39: 333–62.

Kulish, N. (2000). Primary femininity: Clinical advances and theoretical ambiguities. *Journal of the American Psychoanalytic Association* 48: 1355–79.

Kulish, N., and Holtzman, D. (1998). Persephone, the loss of virginity and the female oedipal complex. *International Journal of Psychoanalysis* 79: 57–71.

Lansky, M. (2005). Hidden shame. *Journal of the American Psychoanalytic Association* 53: 865–90.

Lampl De Groot., J. (1927). The evolution of the Oedipus complex in women. *International Journal of Psychoanalysis* 9: 332–45.

Laufer, M. E. (1986). The female Oedipus complex and the relationship to the body. *The Psychoanalytic Study of the Child* 41: 259–76.

Lax, R. (1994). Aspects of primary and secondary genital feelings and anxieties in girls during the preoedipal and early oedipal phases. *Psychoanalytic Quarterly* 63: 271–96.

Lerner, H. (1976). Parental mislabeling of female genitals as a determinant of penis envy and learning inhibitions in women. *Journal of the American Psychoanalytic Association* 24 (Suppl.): 269–83.

Loewald, H. (1978). The waning of the Oedipus complex. *Journal of the American Psychoanalytic Association* 27: 751–75.

Mayer, E. L. (1985). Everybody must be just like me: Observations on female castration anxiety. *International Journal of Psychoanalysis* 66: 331–47.

Morrison, A. (1989). *Shame: The Underside of Narcissism.* Hillsdale, NJ: Analytic Press.

O'Connor, N., and Ryan, J. (1993). *Wild Desires and Mistaken Identities.* New York: Columbia University Press.

Person, E. (1980). Sexuality as the mainstay of identity: Psychoanalytic perspectives. In *Women: Sex and Sexuality,* eds. C. R. Stimpson and E. R. Person. Chicago: University of Chicago Press.

Riviere, J. (1929). Womanliness as masquerade. *International Journal of Psychoanalysis* 10: 303–13.

Rubin, G. (1975), The traffic in women: Notes on the "political economy" of sex. In *Toward an Anthropology of Women,* ed. R. Reiter. New York: Monthly Review Press.

Rubin, L. (1983). *Intimate Strangers.* New York: Harper & Row.

Schafer, R. (1974), Problems in Freud's psychology of women. *Journal of the American Psychoanalytic Association* 22: 459–85.

Schalin, L.J. (1989). On phallicism: Developmental aspects, neutralization, sublimation and defensive phallicism. *Scandinavian Review* 12: 38–57.

Steyn, L. (2009). Is feminine masochism a concept worth reviving? *International Journal of Psychoanalysis* 90: 867–82.

Symonds, A. (1971). Phobias after marriage: Women's declaration of dependence. *American Journal of Psychoanalysis* 31: 144–52.

Torok, M. (1970). The significance of penis envy in women. In *Female Sexuality: New Psychoanalytic Views,* ed. J. Chasseguet-Smirgel. London: Karnac, 135–70.

Tyson, P. (1994). Bedrock and beyond: An examination of the clinical utility of contemporary theories of female psychology. *Journal of the American Psychoanalytic Association* 42: 447–67.

Wolf, N. (1997). *Promiscuities.* New York: Random House.

Zak de Goldstein, R. (1984). The dark continent and its enigmas. *International Journal of Psychoanalysis* 65: 179–89.

ELEVEN

Analysts Who Have Sexual Relations with Their Patients: The Central Role of Masochism

Marvin Margolis, MD, PhD

Masochism is of primary importance in understanding analysts and patients who have become involved in sexual boundary violations. These tragic misalliances destroy reputations and lives and negatively impact the entire psychoanalytic community. Perhaps most importantly is the loss to the patient of an opportunity to gain understanding and relief. Many such patients and others in the community will never again seek out psychoanalysis as a remedy for their psychic pain. Their trust and hope have been destroyed. Therefore, it is imperative that we seek a greater understanding of these catastrophic clinical occurrences. I will base this primarily on my clinical treatment of patients and analysts and in the interest of confidentiality will present aggregate clinical experiences in a schematic summary form. While I refer to analysts, much of what I have to say applies to psychotherapists, as well.

I will attempt to describe a broad spectrum of cases that share many common features especially as regards the issue of masochism. The clinical details are based on multiple experiences. No single case can be inferred from this data. Patients and analysts are never simply masochistic. Therefore, to just isolate out that clinical issue would present data that would be misleading and incomplete. Masochism in the case of sexual boundary violators and their patients is almost always interwoven with narcissism, super ego pathology and often a desperate neediness, all of which may also be embedded in individuals who have many strengths, talents and virtues.

Most of my experience is based on female patients and unethical male analysts. However, with the steady rise in the number of women candidates and analysts, they are also increasingly involved in sexual boundary violations; same sex involvements are also rising in frequency for both male and female analysts. Analysts and candidates of all theoretical persuasion are prone to sexual boundary violations. Finally, there is no evidence that training analysts are any more susceptible to this problem than other graduate analysts and candidates.

We are dealing with a small group of analysts, perhaps 5 percent of our membership, who have done great harm to their patients, themselves, their colleagues, and to psychoanalysis itself. It was their responsibility to analyze their patients and not become sexually involved. Some colleagues feel that every woman analysand would be vulnerable to sexual boundary violation. In its essence this point of view is, at best, patronizing and, at its worst, blatantly sexist. My experience is that every female patient would not be available to the advances of such analysts. Finally, while the responsibility entirely belongs to the analyst, there is a degree of complicity. I will try to describe under what conditions this complicity may occur.

It is likely that in most cases the analyst and patient become sexually involved with each other because of complex determinants stemming from their own histories. This fatal attraction deserves special study. The malignant collusion may often rest on recognition of significant similarities of the analyst and patient to significant people in their respective traumatic childhoods. Oftentimes, this is a singular event for both parties. Some of these cases are certainly treatments that are unworkable and might require early termination and transfer. Others, with adequate consultation/supervision, can have a favorable outcome. It is especially tragic that most of these patients, despite the severity of their pathology, could have been successfully analyzed. In fact, many of these patients were talented and promising clinicians. Some even had hopes of becoming psychoanalysts, and a few have become psychoanalysts.

I will now try to describe the course of development of this type of clinical tragedy. While there is no typical pathway, there are some common features. The analyst is male, clinically experienced and especially drawn to the treatment of challenging cases with which he has had some considerable success. He often is charismatic, likes to please others and craves admiration. The analyst often has been in leadership roles both locally and nationally, and he may have made significant contributions to the literature. Frequently, he has been in a particularly vulnerable state because of recent losses, whether as a result of divorce, death or poor health of self or a family member. Most importantly the analyst has a tendency to experiment with parameters, feeling that by virtue of his experience and authority, he can step outside of the usual technical restraints. The psychology of the exception is relevant to both analyst and patient, especially as it relates to their claim to special privileges due them because they have experienced significant deprivation and losses in their early lives.

The patient is deeply depressed, may be suicidal and is often a very needy person with few close friends. The patient often has a history of past failed treatments and may have been sexually involved with a previous therapist. She is often a candidate or mental health practitioner and usually has a troubled marriage and a history of childhood trauma which may include incest. Her parents also had a troubled marriage and were neglectful. In childhood, the patient may have been frequently and severely beaten by her father, who may also have encouraged rule breaking and anti-social behavior.

The analyst's narcissistic needs drive his seductive attentiveness which quickly wins over his new patient who feels deeply understood and listened to for the first time in her life. The patient begins to feel hopeful. These analysts, from the onset of the treatment, are often self-disclosing, overly helpful and often gossip about colleagues in their psychoanalytic institute. The analysis is usually flawed from the onset, according to these analysands. This is not usually acknowledged by the analyst. He may have become interested in recent psychoanalytic literature that speaks of the value of self-disclosure of love and even sexual attraction towards the patient in the grievously mistaken notion that his confession would help his patient feel better about herself as a woman and help her be more comfortable in her sexuality. The patient feels gratified and privileged, and idealizes the analyst, to whom she is strongly attracted. She begins to have sexual fantasies about the analyst; a highly eroticized transference and countertransference is soon in place. For many months, this treatment continues with minimal analysis of transference, sexual history, current fantasies or the events of early childhood. Often patients divert their transference feelings towards the analyst into destructive sadomasochistic liaisons outside of the analysis, an action which is unrecognized as a transference displacement. The treatment continues, and the patient's depression, anxiety and somatic problems increase as the patient's condition continues to deteriorate. The analyst begins to feel helpless; he is troubled by his lack of success but has no idea why this is the case—he does not seek consultation. The analyst may have a history of seeking consultation and presenting difficult cases to clinical peer groups to which he has belonged for years, but the analyst cannot present this case for group reaction because he feels so unsuccessful and fears being considered incompetent.

The analyst interprets the failing treatment as a signal to further alter his technique in favor of a more personal, gratifying interaction, even offering affection, hugs, and occasional kisses which some patients have all along demanded as signs of the analyst's affection and support. Other patients may be initially shocked that the analyst would initiate such a relationship. Soon, both analyst and patient are trapped. They are caught in a predicament that no longer even resembles a treatment. Both may begin to feel in love. It soon evolves into an exciting and all-absorbing love that can have addictive features.

The patient may be vibrant and seductive. The analyst may feel more sexually alive than he has for a long while. There will be periods of rapturous excitement which alternate with feelings of rejection and despair. Judgment and reality testing gradually vanish as the intoxication peaks. Normal love is not so devoid of reality considerations. The analyst may feel convinced that this is love and dismisses considerations of transference and countertransference. In the down periods, dark, depressive feelings take over. However, the sexual experience may be very powerfully gratifying. The couple gradually drifts into a fuller sexual involvement. The analyst's own marriage begins to be further troubled as his wife reacts to his emotional absence. Oftentimes, the analyst's sexuality may not be robust. He may have difficulty in achieving an erection. His sexuality is often perverse and hurtful physically to the patient. He may not achieve orgasm. The patient may feel that it is her problem that the analyst is not satisfied sexually. He may not allow kissing or intercourse, as if oral or anal sexual acts do not count as love-making.

Occasionally, the therapist prematurely terminates the case and attempts to establish a sexual relationship with the patient outside of the treatment relationship. At this early point, a few back off realizing that they have erred grievously and seek an exit. Sometimes this situation is mediated by an Ethics Committee. These are often the cases in which the sexual boundary violation is of short duration; some analysts are truly remorseful, and accept full responsibility. These cases are most likely to do well in a rehabilitation program.

Unfortunately, many analysts get trapped in this fatal entanglement for months or years, oftentimes because of their inability to work with the patient's masochism and underlying aggression in the transference. Nor can they consciously acknowledge their own growing anger at the patient. The patient's anger at the betrayal is also largely unconscious. This painful clinical impasse also serves their mutual need for punishment for their tabooed sexual behavior by their sadistic superegos. Both obscure this clinical reality with talk of love and possibly a future together. This will not happen and leads only to further anger and hopelessness. They may try to curtail their sexual relationship and convert this into a "friendship." They may consciously feel that they have become each other's closest friend, but it rings hollow; the betrayal and emptiness is the true reality. Some analysts seek to bolster the patient's flagging self-confidence by becoming the patient's patient from time to time as if to level the playing field and act as if the patient's therapeutic skills are equivalent to those of the analyst. They are not aware that Ferenczi tried mutual analysis many years ago and soon discarded it. The analyst feels stuck.

The patient's suicidality may be maximal now, and the threat prevents the analyst from stopping the analysis and referring the patient elsewhere. The patient keeps asking: "where is this heading?" The analyst tries vainly to reassure, but both are increasingly aware of the impossibility of a positive resolution. The atmosphere in the consulting room is that of a Greek tragedy unfolding.

In the course of this consuming affair, the patient has become increasingly cut off from spouse and friends. She cannot talk openly about this secret consuming passion. She lies to cover up their trysts which often occur during lengthened sessions at the end of the day. They are both living double lives. Her depression deepens, and physical ailments multiply. Not infrequently, the patients develop medical conditions such as fibromyalgia and experience excruciating pain. The analyst may become involved in seeking medical remedies for his patient's chronic debilitating pain. The sexual affair now has taken over the entire so-called treatment. The analyst may displace the responsibility for the sexual behavior on the patient. The patients often have to ask the analyst whether or not they can have sex that session and may be asked to dispose of the used condoms. This is experienced by the patient as extremely humiliating. These perverse sadomasochistic interactions are more characteristic of analysts who are not remorseful and who have little-to-no potential for rehabilitation.

The analyst may begin to back away by attempting to terminate the case or refer it to a colleague; oftentimes, this meets with rage as the patient feels abandoned. Again, the analyst fears the patient's wrath, as well as her potential for suicide, so he continues their relationship. Some patients are terrified to quit, fearing the analyst's disapproval. Each now becomes more aware of the other's growing ambivalence and disappointment—expressions of anger become even more open. The relationship is falling apart. The patient and analyst may each secretly seek legal consultations. The patient finally quits and seeks other help.

The patient is now far worse off than before the so-called treatment. Her faith in the analyst or therapist and in treatment in general may prevent her from seeking a professional and/or legal remedy. The patient may also hesitate reporting the analyst for fear of hurting him; others fear the analyst will retaliate. With the passage of time, and perhaps as a result of a new, more helpful treatment, she gradually becomes less frightened of her anger, which now can morph into rage. She may now want to hurt the analyst, even destroy him professionally. For some patients, this may have been their unconscious agenda all along. The patient reports her complaint to an Ethics or Assistance Committee. Finally, the analyst recognizes that his career is in grave jeopardy. Information or gossip about their relationship increasingly enters the public arena. After months of a painful adjudication, the analyst is severely sanctioned and may lose his license to practice as well as his society membership. The analyst's sanctions often involve a suspension from his psychoanalytic society and institute from three to five years or suspension for life. This can involve both local and national membership. If he is a training analyst, he may be ordered to immediately interrupt the analysis of candidates and supervision of candidates. The analyst feels guilty and is deeply ashamed. His candidates are shocked, profoundly upset, and often furious.

The career of the analyst is now severely compromised or destroyed. He may become profoundly depressed or addicted, and some will commit suicide out of a deep sense of shame and hopelessness. The analyst may lose his marriage. Patients and analysts may seek legal solutions that provide financial reparations for patients but avoid ethical proceedings; this adds to the cynicism in the community which is increasingly aware of the sexual boundary violation. Some analysts simply resign their society memberships and professional license and thus avoid onerous sanctions by their colleagues. Would this be so common if a more rehabilitative approach were in place? Accepting the sanctions meted out helps the analyst understand how he has hurt and damaged his colleagues by betraying their joint analytic ideals. This acceptance can be the beginning of his long journey back to his professional community. An increasing number of colleagues undergo rehabilitation: reanalysis and supervision which may help to work out some central problems that were never adequately dealt with in previous analyses, but their careers will likely always be under a cloud.

The patient, who is frequently a mental health professional, often cannot return to practice or seek further treatment as her faith in our field has been undermined. She also may now be physically ill and unable to work. She may also lose her marriage. Some seek out analysis again, and this time there is a reasonable result. The support of colleagues, friends and family is usually a powerful factor in helping these ex-patients and their analysts find their way from the brink of despair to a more realistic and hopeful life.

Unfortunately, these sadomasochistic, tragic treatments impact many others beyond the two protagonists. Most colleagues and candidates in the effected psychoanalytic institute also are deeply disturbed, demoralized and traumatized by these events. Patients and potential patients are disheartened. Practice and recruitment of candidates is negatively affected. Psychoanalysis is once again depreciated in the public square.

Although deeply shaken, our national and local psychoanalytic organizations survive these scandals. The analysts and patients involved find it more difficult to recover. It takes very seasoned, skillful clinicians to take on such cases for second analyses or psychotherapies. Fortunately, there are some successes. Psychoanalytic communities also need time to heal; the aftershocks continue for many years. We are in the early phase of studying this healing process and evaluating the varying solutions underway in the societies and institutes of the American Psychoanalytic Association. Thankfully, most analysts no longer deny the existence of such problems. Unfortunately, it is very common and understandable that our colleagues, who are deeply angered by this betrayal, react by ostracizing the unethical colleagues and provide no institutional pathway to restore membership through rehabilitation programs. Many colleagues do not want to consider the possibility of rehabilitation for these analysts. The unethical analyst and sometimes his candidate/mental health patient are now regarded as damaged goods. Some analysts react as if they see no possibility of transformative change through a reanalysis and supervision. Some analysts turn their backs on these colleagues in an effort to deny that they could ever harbor such wishes or have the potential for such unethical behavior. While there are many unethical analysts that merit permanent extrusion, experience demonstrates that most unethical colleagues benefit from rehabilitation. It is essential that these analysts admit their errors and apologize to their patients (who may also merit compensation) and acknowledge the harm they have done to their patient, to their analytic community and to psychoanalysis. This is humiliating and takes courage. This can be the beginning of a long rehabilitation process. Some advocate treatments (usually psychotherapy) other than analysis for those analysts. My experience is that they need a new analysis because major issues were not dealt with in earlier analyses. However, they are often analyzable; we should give analysis another try.

It is equally important to address the conditions that contribute to sexual boundary violations. Analysts and therapists must seek consultation when they have persistent feelings of love and erotic desire for particular patients. This should be discussed with colleagues, not with patients. Greater clarity about the issue of "love" in analysis is required. While we care deeply about our patients; we should be wary of labeling this as love. If the analyst feels it is love, he or she should seek a consultation. The colleagues sought out for consultation should neither be friends, previous therapists or colleagues who would share one's enthusiasm for innovative treatment techniques that advocate self-disclosures of love and desire to ones patients. Ethics education for all mental health practitioners must be a continuous and lifelong responsibility. Even though we can never completely eliminate this problem, there is much that we can do to help colleagues deal more effectively with the potential for sexual boundary violations. Perhaps even more importantly, by studying these tragic cases, we can learn much about improving our general understanding of the psychoanalytic enterprise for all cases.

In summary: I hope that this schematic overview illustrates that masochism is central to the phenomenon of sexual boundary violations. The core of the problem can be seen as residing in unresolved pre-genital conflicts which must be fundamentally addressed before oedipal issues can be effectively analyzed. Both patient and analyst have never been able to fully face the pain of their traumatic past. Masochism organized around very sadistic primitive superego functions masks a deep rage at parents and even the larger society who could not provide the fundamental safety and love which is necessary to develop trust and the ability to love. These are parents who are often role models for lying and dishonesty. The analyst was unable to deeply work with the rage, the profound loneliness and the desperation of his patient, for he has never adequately dealt with these issues in his own previous analysis. With some, it was an inadequate analyst; with others these issues were unconsciously kept out of the analysis by the patient and future analyst. Consequently, faced with cases that mirror his own conflicts, he soon abandons analysis and reacts to the patient's neediness with a pseudo-love that can never satisfy or heal but only frustrate and re-traumatize. The underlying sense of betrayal, sadism, wish for revenge on the part of the patient eventually doom these fatal experiments. The pain and suffering of both escalates despite the partial pleasure allowed some patients by a revengeful destruction of the analyst's career. The ruin of careers, reputation and marriages are the rule. It is not a triumph of their sadistic natures that is so prominent in the end, but rather the masochistic denouement that is the most prominent feature of the end of their mutual clinical involvement. There is often a narcissistic core to their masochistic complaints. I think of Oedipus in his last years. In *Oedipus Rex* we learn of his unwitting murder of his father Laius and subsequent incestuous marriage to his mother Jocasta with whom he had four children. In his youth, as son of the king and queen of Corinth, he had heard of his adoption but not of the particulars. In *Oedipus Rex* there was an unraveling of his past in Thebes where he was now the monarch. Traumatic moments of his early life are now revealed, culminating in the discovery that his biological mother, at the behest of his biological father, had sought his death by abandoning him to a certain death on a mountain top. When this is revealed, his mother runs to her chambers. Oedipus follows in a rage, only to find that she has committed suicide. Overcome by grief over the loss of his wife/mother, and perhaps by guilt as well, he then blinds himself with her broaches; subsequently he is banished from Thebes and, accompanied by his two loyal daughters, is doomed to wander the earth. In *Oedipus at Colonus,* in an outburst of masochistic grandiosity, he exclaims: "Was there ever a man who suffered more in this world?" There is no recognition that he had ruined the lives of his two daughters who have had to accompany and care for their blind father in his exile. Nor does Oedipus demonstrate anything other than anger towards his sons who end their lives killing each other in battle. More importantly, Oedipus now backs away from the central truths of his impulsive, incestuous and arrogant life and spends these final years of exile as a defiant and cruel man living in disgrace and glorifying his painful masochistic existence. It is the challenge of these stubborn, complex masochistic problems that is central to the work of the reanalysis of these patients.

REFERENCES

Celenza, A. (2007). *Sexual Boundary Violations*. Northvale, NJ: Jason Aronson (1995).

Gabbard, G. O., and Lester, E. (1995). *Boundaries and Boundary Violations in Psychoanalysis*. New York: Basic Books.

Gabbard, G. O., and Peltz, M. (2001). Speaking the unspeakable: Institutional reactions to boundary violations by training analysts (COPE Study Group on Boundary Violations). *Journal of the American Psychoanalytic Association* 49: 659–73.

Jacobson, E. (1954). The exceptions: An elaboration of Freud's character study. *Psychoanalytic Study of the Child* 14: 135–54.

Margolis, M. (1994). Incest, erotic countertransference and analyst-analysand boundary violations. *Journal of the American Psychoanalytic Association* 42: 985–89.

——— (1997). Analyst-patient sexual involvement: Clinical experiences and institutional responses. *Psychoanalytic Inquiry* 17: 349–69

———(2009). Meeting the challenges of rehabilitation for boundary violations. *Newsletter of the American Psychoanalyst* 43(2): 25–33.

Roche, P. (1996). *The Oedipus Plays of Sophocles*. New York: A Meridian Book/Penguin Group.

Sandler, A. (2004). Institutional response to boundary violations: The case of Masud Khan. *International Journal of Psychoanalysis* 85: 27–44.

Conclusion

Deanna Holtzman, PhD, and Nancy Kulish, PhD

Masochism is understood, here, as the individual's active pursuit of psychic or physical pain, suffering and humiliation in his or her life. Building on their predecessors, the psychoanalytic thinkers in this collection have provided creative and valuable contributions to current theory and treatment of masochism, certainly one of the most challenging clinical problems we as clinicians face. The contributors in this volume have been in the forefront of bringing forth new understandings of these enigmatic conditions. They demonstrate clearly the means of applying complex but illuminating theories about the origins, meanings and functions of masochism to real-life clinical situations. The generous clinical examples provide immediate and exquisite descriptions of countertransference/transference turmoil and the way out of these Sisyphean dilemmas. These clinical examples help to enhance our armamentarium of pragmatic interventions. We can feel that these authors are our "partners" in our work as they have given us a more organized, cohesive set of ways to think about and deal with behaviors and symptoms that have stymied us and our patients.

We point to the more striking themes which have emerged in this collection in dealing with sadomasochism: First, the traumatic based origins of these phenomena; second, the underlying object relational issues which range from early misalignment and inabilities to soothe the infant through triadic shame and humiliation; third, the better appreciated and recognized role of aggression which fuels the defensive symptomology and character disorders across the masochistic spectrum. We are convinced that the greater the masochism, the greater the pool of sadism that feeds it; fourth, the frequent defensive use of sexuality to cover over sadism or problems of self-cohesion; fifth, the vulnerability of every clinician who works with deeply masochistic patients to being overwhelmed with narcissistic defeat and impotency and accompanying feelings of hatred and shame; sixth, the interesting insight that these patients need to externalize guilt by inducing it in others; seventh, the crucial, empathic emphasis on the adaptive and meaningful nature of masochism for the individual; eighth, how countertransference/transferences take center stage in the therapeutic drama; ninth, the importance for the clinician to be able to maintain equanimity in the face of dramatic challenges posed by the inevitable sadomasochistic interactions that disrupt the therapeutic frame and relationship and, if necessary, to be able to seek consultation with a colleague.

In conclusion, whatever differences exist in their emphases on sexuality, aggression, narcissism, diagnoses, or technique, all of the contributors agree that there are a variety of clinical phenomena in which there seems to be an obligatory relationship between pain and often unconscious pleasure, or put differently, a variety of patients who actively pursue psychic or physical pain, suffering, or humiliation. These ways of living one's life that seem to defy common sense and defy change are profoundly puzzling to the ordinary observer. We think that psychoanalysis and its understandings of unconscious and complex motivations offer one of the only avenues of hope of mitigating such self-propelled and deeply embedded suffering. Our authors have shown us that it is the psychoanalytically informed treatments—psychoanalysis or psychotherapy—that hold out hope, because they alone provide a method of understanding and working through these intense, sadomasochistic dramas that define the work. Such masochistic patients have given up almost all hope for any happiness or cessation of pain; in the analytic situation, they inevitably try to reproduce their despair and to undermine and to destroy their analyst's hope. We are struck by how all of our contributors speak to this question of *analytic hope*; in their different ways they have managed to hold on to their hope and transmit it to their patients and, we believe, to us. Thus, we are no longer condemned to suffer like Sisyphus.

Index

adaptation, masochism as, 61, 87, 104, 135

adolescence, masochism in: Novicks on, 51–73n1; Sugarman on, 29–48

affection, masochism and, 116

aggression: expression of, 38; and masochism, 7, 16–17, 21, 40–41; toddlerhood and, 55

aggressor, seduction of, 151

anal stage, and masochism, 30

analysis. *See* technical and therapeutic implications

analyst: attitudes of, 11–12; and closed and open systems, 65; and masochism, 3, 26, 51, 67, 79, 87, 107, 153; modes of relating for, 129–143n1; moral masochism and, 25; and narcissistic masochism, 116; and open-system functioning, 66; as parent, 89, 109; and sadomasochistic stuckness, 89–101; and sexual boundary violations, 13, 104, 187–195

anger: narcissistic, 113–125n1; and sexual relations with patient, 191. *See also* aggression

anorexia nervosa, 115; masochism in, 146–151; as suicidality, 117

anxiety: and analysis, 140; management of, and masochism, 37, 131

Asch, S. S., 34, 35–36

attachment: disturbed, and masochism, 35, 54; sadomasochistic, 83–86

Azmi, Shabana, 161

B (patient), 89–101

Balsam, R., 92

beating fantasy, 30, 157; aggressive drive and, 41; in childhood, 29; Nick and, 62, 69; projection of, 152

being with, and masochism, 68

Benjamin, J., 161, 165

Bergler, D., 30, 35

Berliner, Bernhard, 116, 124

Bernstein, D., 169

Bion, W. R., 105, 134, 137, 139

Blum, Harold P., 145–159

Bobby (patient), 33–34, 35, 36, 40

body image: female shame and, 171; sadomasochistic stuckness and, 95

borderline personality organization, and masochism, 18–19; prognosis in, 24

boundary violations: analyst and, 104, 187–195, 13; factors affecting, 193; mother and, 84

brain trap, 55

Branchaft, B., 124

Brandschaft, Bernard, 5

Brenman, M., 116

bulimia: as suicidality, 117; trauma and, 146

Burgner, M., 30

Busch, F., 32

castration anxiety: and masochism, 104, 158; and perverse masochism, 153

change, avoidance of, 105, 107; Joseph on, 129, 133; masochism and, 108; narcissistic rage and, 118; sadomasochistic stuckness and, 99–100

character structure: masochistic, 77–88n1; narcissistic-masochistic, 80

Chassegeut-Smirgel, J., 168

childhood, masochism in, as self-regulatory disorder, 29–48
children: and masochism, 72; and narcissistic masochism, 121–122
Chused, J. F., 41
closed-system functioning, 52–53; definition of, 52; developmental underpinnings and derivatives of, 54–59; and open system, 70; technical approaches to, 59–65
Coen, Stanley J., 41, 89–101
Colarusso, Calvin A., 33
competitiveness, masochism and, 109
contentment, and interpretation, 139
control. *See* omnipotence
Cooper, A., 37, 80, 104, 106, 114
Cooper, S. H., 105
countertransference: and interpretation, 132, 139; and masochism, 3, 9–10, 26, 85–86; and narcissism, 120; Segal on, 130–132; and sexual relations with patient, 189
cutting, 35, 156; as suicidality, 117

death drive: clinical example of, 141–143; confrontation with, 132; and masochism, 131; narcissism and, 135
defenses: absent desire as, 162, 167; negative therapeutic reaction, 25; omnipotence as, 71; self psychology on, 123
denial: closed-system functioning and, 52; omnipotence and, 38
dependency, and masochism, 20, 21, 99, 130
depressive-masochistic personality disorder, 20–21, 113; prognosis in, 23
desire, women and, 161; mother and, 164; negation of, 165; oedipal defeat and, 167
development: gender and, 165–167; self psychology on, 123
developmental images, and masochism, 68
developmental lag, 32
DeVito, E., 54

Dimen, M., 161
divorce, and narcissistic masochism, 121
Doidge, N., 55
Dracula theme, 176–177, 178

E (patient), 141–143
early object relations, and masochism, 5–6
ego psychology, 114
Elise, Dianne, 161–183n11
emotional muscle, omnipotence and, 67–68
environment, and masochism, 41–43
envy: and analysis, 138; masochism and, 109, 117
externalization, closed-system functioning and, 62–63

failure of treatment, as narcissistic structure, 82
failure to thrive: masochistic submission and, 162, 164, 181; term, 182n2
family system, externalizations in, 62
father: and adolescence, 54; analyst as, 109; Freud on, 30; and masochism, 42–43, 46, 57, 59, 84, 92; and narcissistic masochism, 116, 121; and toddlerhood, 55; treatment and, 67; and women and submission, 164
father figures, and masochism, 68
feeling with, and masochism, 68
Feldman, Michael, 131, 132–133
feminine masochism, 179–181; term, 180
Fenichel, O., 31, 104
Fischer, N., 114
Freud, Anna, 52, 157
Freud, Sigmund: on feminine masochism, 179; on masochism, 2, 30, 44, 78, 129; on negative therapeutic reaction, 25; on Oedipus complex, 162, 166; on phallic narcissism, 169; on shame, 168; on superego, 33; on women, 161
functional dystonia, 55
fusion urges: and analysis, 142; and masochism, 35–36, 96

Gabbard, Glen, 64, 103–111
Gabriella (patient), 37–38
gender: and diagnosis of masochism, 22, 103; masochism and, 161–183n11
generalization, 63
Glick, Robert Alan, 77–88n1, 113
grandiosity. *See* omnipotence
Gray, P., 32
Green, André, 22, 130, 135, 141
guilt. *See* unconscious guilt

hatred, and therapy, 12
helplessness: as addictive, 131–132, 135; and analysis, 137; and sexual relations with patient, 189; as trauma, 52. *See also* shame
heterosexual role development, 165–166, 183n6
holding, and understanding, 121
Holtzman, Deanna, 1–14, 163, 164, 174, 197–198
homeostasis, need for, 64

imprisonment, sense of, 130
independent therapeutic work, and masochism, 71
infancy, and closed-system functioning, 54–55
interpretation, interpretive interventions: Bion on, 139; and countertransference, 132; and masochism, 139, 153; and open system, 66; and suicidality, 25

James, William, 130
Jones, E., 167
Joseph, B., 9, 129, 130–132, 132–133, 135
jouissance, 105

Kate (patient), 174–179
Kennedy, H., 30
Kernberg, Otto, 15–26, 103
Klein, Melanie, 105, 129
Kohut, Heinz, 114, 122, 124
Krafft-Ebing, R., 78
Kulish, Nancy, 1–14, 163, 164, 174, 197–198

L (patient), 106–109

Lacan, J., 105
lateness, 81–82
Lawrence (patient), 38–39, 42–43
Lerner, H., 182
listening: for omnipotent beliefs, 61–62; and transference, 119
lived experiences, self psychology on, 123
Loewald, H. W., 163–164, 178, 181
love relations: masochism and, 51, 58, 69, 72, 86; perverse masochism and, 152. *See also* marriage

Maleson, F., 113
Margolis, Marvin, 187–195
Markman, Henry, 129–143n1
marriage: masochism and, 11, 72, 82–83, 106; masochistic submission and, 174–179, 180–181; narcissistic rage and, 115, 117, 118. *See also* love relations
masochism, 1–14, 197–198; analyzability of, 16, 18, 31, 151; Blum on, 145–159; Coen on, 89–101; contemporary understandings of, 3–9, 15–17; definition of, 1, 2, 3–4, 78, 113, 145; developmental origins of, 4–9; diagnosis of, 3–4, 22–26, 114; Elise on, 161–183n11; Gabbard on, 103–111; history of study of, 78, 113; Kernberg on, 15–26, 103; manifestations of, 81–86, 145; Markman on, 129–143n1; as multiply determined, 6, 103–111, 116; Novicks on, 51–73n1; as pervasive, 15, 77–78, 103, 114, 145; prognosis in, 23–24; sadism and, 51; and sexual relations with patient, 187–195; structural features of, 33–43; Sugarman on, 29–48. *See also* sadomasochism
masochistic character structure, 77–88n1
masochistic experience: clinical examples of, 136–143; motivation and, 135; varieties of, 129–143n1
masochistic pathology, levels of, 17–22
masochistic phenomena, versus narcissistic, 135

mastery: and masochism, 104; need for, 64

mental structure, and masochism, 32–43

Meyers, D. I., 78, 113

money, attitudes toward, and masochism, 83–84

moral masochism, 25, 78, 113

Morrison, A., 168

mother: and adolescence, 54; analyst as, 89; and anorexia, 146–149; and masochism, 36, 41–43, 46, 54, 57, 58, 59, 83–86, 154; and masochistic submission in women, 162, 163, 170–174, 176, 177, 178; and narcissistic masochism, 114, 116, 141; and oedipal development, 165; and omnipotence, 40; and pain seeking, 35, 54; therapy and, 67, 69; and toddlerhood, 55

movies, as therapeutic tool, 85

N (patient), 136–141

narcissism: and marriage, 175, 178, 180; and masochism, 2, 5–6, 19, 21, 24, 36–40, 80, 104, 114; versus masochistic phenomena, 135; phallic, 169; and sexual relations with patient, 189; and submission, 178

narcissistic-masochistic character structure, 80; clinical example of, 141–143

narcissistic rage, 113–125n1; clinical example of, 115–123; self psychology on, 123–125

needs: closed-system functioning and, 61; denial of, 130

negative therapeutic reaction, 9, 34–36; and unconscious guilt, 25

neurotic personality organization, and masochism, 20

Nick (patient), 51, 53; in adolescence, 59; in infancy, 54–55; in oedipal stage, 57–58; in school age, 58; therapy with, 59–73; in toddlerhood, 55–57

Novick, Jack, 30, 32, 38, 39, 51–73n1; on omnipotence, 40; on pre-oedipal stage, 45; on self-regulation, 45; on stuckness, 90; on superego, 46; on toddlerhood, 40

Novick, Kerry Kelly, 30, 32, 38, 39, 51–73n1; on omnipotence, 40; on pre-oedipal stage, 45; on self-regulation, 45; on stuckness, 90; on superego, 46; on toddlerhood, 40

oedipal defeat: double, 165; and shame, 162, 168–170

oedipal stage, and masochism, 30, 33, 57–58

Oedipus complex: emphasis on, 31–32, 37; and women and submission, 162, 163–167

Oedipus plays, 193

omnipotence: adolescence and, 59; analysis and, 140; closed-system functioning and, 52, 61–62; delusion of, 38; and emotional muscle, 67–68; and fantasy, 104; and love relations, 69; and masochism, 2, 37–40, 45, 51; narcissistic-masochistic character structure and, 80; parents and, 62; school age and, 58; and therapy, 107; toddlerhood and, 56

open system: and closed system, 70; definition of, 52; fostering, 66–73; as goal, 65

Ornstein, Anna, 113–125n1

P (patient), 146–151

pain. *See* suffering

parents. *See* father; mother

pathogenic models, reconsideration of, 31–32

patient-analyst sexual relations, 187–195; development of, 188–189; effects of, 191–192; factors affecting, 193; incidence of, 188

personality structure, and analyzability of masochism, 16

perverse masochism, clinical example of, 151–158

perversion: encapsulated, 152; term, 151

phallic narcissism, 169

phallic stage, and masochism, 57–58

Phillip (patient), 39–40
pity, countertransference and, 26
pleasure, and suffering: and analysis, 130; clinical example of, 82–83; and shame, 171, 172
pleasure principle, and theory on masochism, 114
pre-oedipal stages, masochism in, 29–30
primary masochism, 16
projective identification: and analyst, 138; term, 63
protomasochistic pathology, 29–30; versus masochistic, 32, 34
psychoanalytic self psychology, on sadomasochism, 123–125
psychotherapist. *See* analyst
psychotherapy. *See* technical and therapeutic implications

R (patient), 151–158
rapprochement subphase, of separation–individuation, 155
reality: closed-system functioning and, 52, 53; and sexual relations with patient, 190; therapy and, 61
regression: analyst and, 92, 100; sadomasochistic stuckness and, 93–94
relational masochism, 103, 108
representational world, and masochism, 34–36
resentment, countertransference and, 26
respect, and closed-system functioning, 60
responsibility: feminine oedipal development and, 164; masochism and, 108; and sexuality, 173, 174
Rosen, Irwin, 103
Rosenfeld, H. A., 35, 40, 133–134, 140, 142

Sacher-Masoch, Leopold von, 78, 103
sadism, 1; and conflict, 146; indirect, 116; and masochism, 51
sadomasochism: versus depressive-masochism, 113; Novicks on, 51–73n1; psychoanalytic self

psychology on, 123–125; and self-organization, 133; term, 1, 51. *See also* masochism
sadomasochistic stuckness, 2, 89–101, 105, 107, 130, 131, 136, 140; and sexual relations with patient, 189, 190; submission and, 177
Sally (patient), 113
Sara (patient), 170–174
Sarah (patient), 29–30, 35–36, 47
Schafer, R., 77–78, 179
Schalin, L. J., 169
Schneidman, E. S., 117
school age, and masochism, 58
secrets, masochism and, 87
seduction of aggressor, 151
Segal, Hannah, 130, 132
self-criticism, 105
self-harming symptoms, 12; clinical example of, 115–123; narcissistic rage and, 113–125n1; and pleasure, 16
self-organization, pathological models of, 133–134, 138, 140
self psychology, on sadomasochism, 123–125
self-reflection, 11
self-regulation, and masochism: aim of, 53; and internal conflict, 70; Novicks on, 51–73n1; Sugarman on, 29–48
self-sacrifice, 22, 157; analyst and, 104–105; and anorexia, 149
sexual boundary violations: analyst and, 13, 104, 187–195; factors affecting, 193; mother and, 84
sexuality, and masochism, 2, 6–7; versus aggression, 41; avoidance in therapy, 91, 94, 97, 170; oedipal phase and, 58; perverse masochism, 151–158; responsibility and, 173, 174; shame and, 171–172
shame: definition of, 168; and masochistic submission in women, 161–183n11; oedipal defeat and, 162, 168–170
siblings, and masochism, 54, 56, 97
single-track developmental theory, critique of, 64
Sisyphus, 1

sleep, during analysis, 107–108
soul blindness, 59, 62
soul murder, 83
Steiner, J., 133
Stern, D., 54
Steyn, L., 180
Stoller, Robert, 16
Stolorow, R., 114
stuckness. *See* sadomasochistic
    stuckness
sublimation, masochism and, 22
submission, masochistic: clinical
    examples of, 170–179; women and,
    161–183n11
substance abuse: masochism and, 51,
    59, 62; as suicidality, 117
suffering: and analysis, 137, 139;
    closed-system functioning and, 52;
    drive toward, and analysis, 129; and
    masochism, 15; need for, clinical
    example of, 82–83; sharing, nature
    of, 120
Sugarman, Alan, 29–48
suicidality, 12; clinical example of,
    115–123; closed-system functioning
    and, 60; interpretation of, 25;
    mother and, 84; narcissistic rage
    and, 113–125n1; and therapy, 24
superego, and masochism, 15, 33–34,
    46, 129
Symonds, A., 181

technical and therapeutic implications:
    and anorexia, 151; basic
    assumptions of, 63–64; and closed-
    system functioning, 59–65; goal of
    treatment, 65, 79, 132; guiding
    dynamic constructs for, 80;
    Kernberg on, 22–26; and
    masochism, 9–13, 52, 87, 106–109;
    modes of relating with masochistic
    experience, 129–143n1; and open-
    system functioning, 66–73; and
    sadomasochistic stuckness, 89–101;
    timeframe of therapy, 9, 52, 122, 135
termination: L and, 109; Nick and,
    70–72; Sarah and, 35; and sexual
    relations with patient, 190; timing
    of, 122

theory, on masochism, 2–3, 79–80; and
    diagnosis, 114; women and, 163–170
therapeutic alliance, and open system,
    66, 67
therapeutic attitude, shifting, 95
therapeutic dialogue: definition of,
    125n1; in narcissistic rage, 115, 118
therapeutic implications. *See* technical
    and therapeutic implications
toddlerhood: and closed-system
    functioning, 55–57; and
    development of masochism, 40
transference: analyst and, 119; and
    closed-system functioning, 59;
    management of, 24; and masochism,
    9–10, 23; and masochistic
    submission, 177; and narcissism,
    119; omnipotence and, 39; and
    open-system functioning, 66, 67;
    and sexual relations with patient,
    189; split, 36; toddlerhood and, 56
Transference Focused Psychotherapy,
    18, 25
trauma: change as, 133; definition of,
    146; effects of, 158; helplessness as,
    52; and masochism, 4–5, 17–18, 80,
    114, 145–159; mastery and, 104; and
    narcissistic rage, 124; and self-
    organization, 134
trichotillomania, 37–38
Tyson, P., 32, 33, 41, 45, 46
Tyson, R. L., 33

unconscious guilt: analysis of, 87;
    Freud on, 2; and masochism, 8–9,
    20, 30, 33, 80, 156; negative
    therapeutic reaction and, 25
understanding, narcissistic rage and,
    120–121

Valenstein, A. F., 30

Waelder, R., 44
White (patient), 115–123
Williams, Paul, 134
Winnicott, Donald, 121
Wolf, N., 161
women: and diagnosis of masochism,
    22, 103; masochism and, 161–183n11

working together, and masochism, 68–69

Wurmser, L., 59, 62, 70

Zerbe, K. J., 146

About the Contributors

Harold P. Blum, MD, is a training and supervising analyst at the Institute for Psychoanalytic Education, affiliated with New York University and clinical professor of psychiatry, New York University School of Medicine. He is the past editor of *The Journal of the American Psychoanalytic Association* and past vice president of the International Psychoanalytic Association. He is the author of several books and more than 160 professional papers.

Stanley J. Coen, MD, is a training and supervising analyst and senior associate director for academic affairs at the Columbia University Center for Psychoanalytic Training and Research, clinical professor of psychiatry at the Columbia University College of Physicians and Surgeons, and a member of several psychoanalytic editorial boards. The author of three books and many articles, he has published extensively on problems in clinical psychoanalysis and psychoanalytic literary criticism.

Dianne Elise, PhD, is a personal and supervising analyst and member of the faculty at the Psychoanalytic Institute of Northern California and a training analyst at the International Psychoanalytic Association. Dr. Elise is associate editor of *Studies in Gender and Sexuality* and a past editorial board member for *The Journal of the American Psychoanalytic Association*. She has published extensively on issues of gender and female sexuality. She has a private practice in Oakland, California.

Glen O. Gabbard, MD, is professor of psychiatry at SUNY Upstate Medical University in Syracuse, New York, clinical professor of psychiatry at Baylor College of Medicine in Houston, and training and supervising analyst at the Center for Psychoanalytic Studies in Houston. He is former joint editor-in-chief of *The International Journal of Psychoanalysis*. He is the author or editor of twenty-seven books, including *Love and Hate in the Analytic Setting*, *Textbook of Psychoanalysis*, *Boundaries and Boundary Violations in Psychoanalysis*, and *Psychodynamic Psychiatry in Clinical Practice*, *4th Edition*.

Robert Alan Glick, MD, is professor of clinical psychiatry, Columbia University College of Physicians and Surgeons, former director of the Columbia University Center for Psychoanalytic Training and Research

(1997–2007) and training and supervising psychoanalyst at the Columbia University Center. He was former associate editor for education of *The Journal of the American Psychoanalytic Association*. Dr. Glick has edited a series of volumes on the psychoanalytic theory of affects, and published numerous chapters and articles on psychoanalytic and psychiatric education.

Deanna Holtzman, PhD, is a training and supervising analyst and past president of the Michigan Psychoanalytic Institute. She is an adjunct professor in the Department of Psychiatry, School of Medicine at Wayne State University and an adjunct professor of psychology at the University of Detroit. She is the president of the Sigmund Freud Archives, Inc., and has coauthored two books with Nancy Kulish.

Otto F. Kernberg, M.D.F.A.P.A, is director of the Personality Disorders Institute at The New York Presbyterian Hospital, Westchester Division, professor of psychiatry at the Weill Medical College of Cornell University, and past president of the International Psychoanalytic Association. He is also training and supervising analyst of the Columbia University Center for Psychoanalytic Training and Research. He is the author of thirteen books and coauthor of twelve others, and numerous articles on a wide range of topics including diagnostic issues in clinical psychiatry and psychoanalysis, group processes, and the therapeutic process.

Nancy Kulish, PhD, is a training and supervising analyst and past president of the Michigan Psychoanalytic Institute. She is an adjunct professor in the Department of Psychiatry, School of Medicine at Wayne State University and an adjunct professor of psychology at the University of Detroit. She has coauthored two books with Deanna Holtzman and published numerous articles on transference/countertransference, gender, and female sexuality.

Marvin Margolis, MD, PhD, is a training and supervising analyst at the Michigan Psychoanalytic Institute and a clinical associate professor of psychiatry at Wayne State University School of Medicine. He is past chair of the ethics committee, past chairman of the Board of Professional Standards, and past president of the American Psychoanalytic Association. His research interests include ethics, sexual boundary violations and rehabilitation, parent-child incest, masochistic perversions, mythology, and dreams.

Henry Markman, MD, is a training and supervising analyst, and member of the faculty at the San Francisco Center for Psychoanalysis and training analyst at the Psychoanalytic Institute of Northern California. He has published articles on the treatment of adolescents, aesthetic experience in psychoanalysis, metaphor as theory, neo-Kleinian contributions to technique, and music and psychoanalysis.

Jack Novick, PhD, graduated from the Hampstead Clinic in 1969 and the British Psycho-Analytic Institute in 1971. He was on the faculty of the Hampstead Clinic from 1970–1977. He is a child and adult training and supervising analyst of the International Psychoanalytic Association and serves on numerous psychoanalytic institute faculties. With Kerry Kelly Novick, he has published many papers and four books on a wide variety of psychoanalytic topics.

Kerry Kelly Novick is a child, adolescent, and adult psychoanalyst who graduated from the Hampstead Clinic (Anna Freud Centre) in 1970, and was a staff member from 1970–1977. A child and adult training and supervising analyst of the International Psychoanalytic Association, she is on the faculties of numerous psychoanalytic institutes. She has published many papers, and written four books with Jack Novick on a wide variety of psychoanalytic topics.

Anna Ornstein, MD, is a retired professor of child psychiatry of University of Cincinnati and currently lecturer in psychiatry, Harvard Medical School, Cambridge, Massachusetts, and supervising analyst, Boston Psychoanalytic Institute. She has over one hundred publications ranging from papers on the interpretive process in psychoanalysis, to child-centered family treatment, to the survival and recovery of extreme conditions.

Alan Sugarman, PhD, is a training and supervising psychoanalyst and a child and adolescent supervising psychoanalyst at the San Diego Psychoanalytic Society and Institute. He is also a clinical professor of psychiatry at the University of California, San Diego, and maintains a private practice in La Jolla, California. Dr. Sugarman is widely published, mostly focusing on the application of psychoanalytic developmental thinking to diagnosis and treatment.